HOLISTIC AROMATHERAPY FOR BODYWORKERS

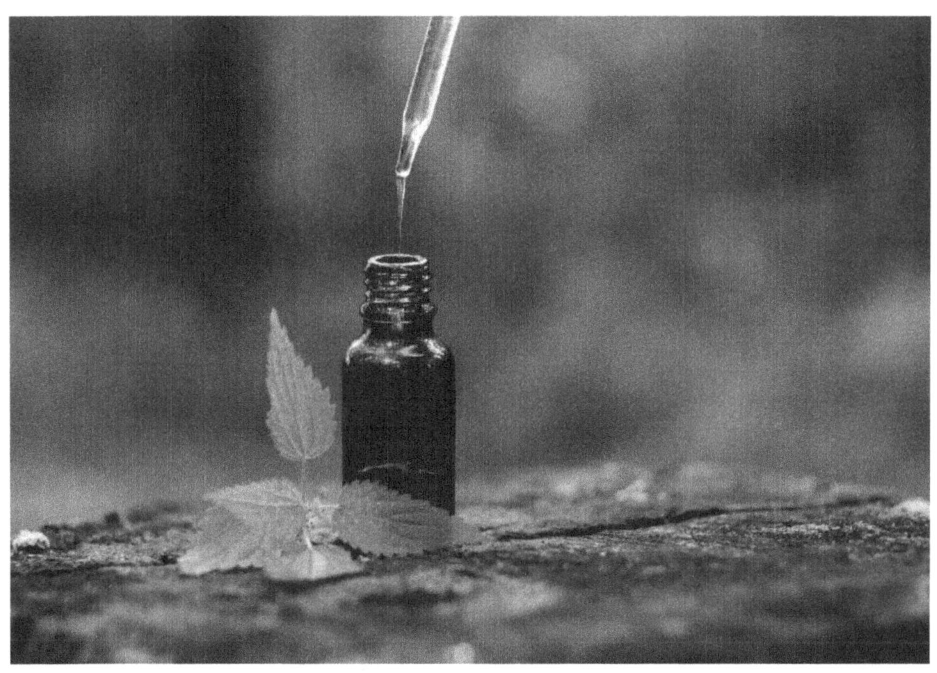

FERNANDA SANTIAGO

Notice of Liability

The author has made an effort to ensure the information in this manual is accurate. The author will not be held liable for any damages due to the instruction or information contained within.

*Aromatherapy is a Complementary Alternative Medicine (CAM) and is not used by any form to replace medical care if necessary. Do not use essential oils internally or undiluted on the skin. Always test a small amount of the essential oil first for sensitivity or allergic reaction. The FDA has not evaluated the statements in this publication. No claims are made as to any medicinal value of the oils or any products mentioned. The information presented here is for educational purposes of traditional uses and is not intended to diagnose, treat, cure, or prevent any disease. You are responsible for understanding the safe application of these products. If you have any questions, please call or email us for further information.

Praise from our Readers

"I picked up my first aromatherapy chart at 14 years old, in a new age church bookstore. As I peered over the glossy laminate, my mind was amazed at what I read, that all these essential oils were like magical keys that could unlock boundless benefits to my brain and body. It felt magical and sacred. Instantly I was hooked, enrolling in my first aromatherapy class and starting a brand new pathway that would lead to my career of choice. I've currently been a massage therapist for 18 years and aromatherapy has been an integral part of my practice the entire time. From services like chakra alignment and vagus nerve massage to curating my own scrubs and topicals with the desired essential oils, the power of plants never ceases to amaze me. I tell all of my clients jokingly, "If you don't like scented things, you probably don't want to come to my spa."

Fast forward over 20 years later to meeting Fernanda virtually via the founder of Badass Bodyworkers, Rebecca Brumfield, who spoke highly of her and thought we would really get along. But it wasn't her infectious smile or charming demeanor that made me like her, it was her passion. Her enthusiasm for her respected niches came through in her voice as she spoke and her dedication to ethically sourced ingredients and tools was apparent. I instantly became fond of her and wanted to learn more.

So when I received the invitation to take one of her virtual continuing education classes, I jumped at the opportunity. When you've had a solid 23 years dabbling in aromatherapy, you don't expect to learn much more but I was so wrong. The information she shares really makes you think about your consumption and appreciate the beauty in using the Earth's most precious gifts, the plants.

Aromatherapy has the power to do almost everything. The healing capabilities are endless and it is because of the dedication to the craft from women like Fernanda that the industry will hopefully receive more funding and research dedicated to this ancient practice.

I speak to Fernanda every day at this point. Her wisdom continues to astound me. These are the kinds of teachers we need in this world. Teachers that are devoted to maintaining the wisdom of our ancestors for generations to come.

So as you proceed in reading, take some pauses to really think about the gift of plant based healing and hopefully you fall in love with the practice of using aromatherapy even more. Thank you Fernanda, for teaching a whole new generation of practitioners to unlock the magic of the Earth's remedies once again."

-Jessica York LMT, CL, BCTMB

"Fernanda's passion for herbalism and aromatherapy shines through in her book, Holistic Aromatherapy for Bodyworkers. She makes it easy for newcomers to aromatherapy to not only learn about the properties of each plant and herb, but also to be able to use her book as a guide as they learn to incorporate it into their bodywork practice. Her mix of history of using herbs as medicine, scientific background of each plant, a physio-social connection to essential oils, and how-to structure is what makes her book a fun and engaging read! You'll be excited to put your new knowledge to action!"

-Susan Good,

Owner-Latitude Massage

"Holistic Aromatherapy for Bodyworkers is a truly exceptional textbook that delves deep into the world of aromatherapy, offering a comprehensive and insightful exploration of this ancient practice. From its historical origins to its modern applications, this book provides a thorough understanding of aromatherapy's principles, techniques, and benefits. It seamlessly blends the artistry of scent with the scientific principles behind aromatherapy, making it accessible to both newcomers and seasoned practitioners. The author provides detailed guidelines on how to use essential oils safely and effectively. This book is a must-have resource for anyone interested in the practice of aromatherapy." -

Michelle Roos,

LMT, Owner- Cupping Canada

Dedication

To my teachers, whose wisdom guided my steps,

To my mentors, whose patience nurtured my growth,

To my students, whose curiosity fueled my passion,

And to all who have supported me on this aromatic journey,

I extend my deepest gratitude and heartfelt appreciation.

Special thanks to my father,

Whose lessons in healing plants paved the way,

Whose encouragement ignited the flame,

And whose love continues to illuminate my path.

This book is dedicated to you all,

May its pages be infused with the essence of our shared journey.

With love and gratitude,

Fernanda

Forward

You're driving along a country road and suddenly you catch a whiff… a scent that drenches your consciousness with long lost nostalgic memories, the smell of fresh spring cut grass evokes strong emotional responses and the thought of your mother's cooking brings back countless childhood souvenirs. Our sense of smell is not only linked to emotions and memory, but also completes our sense of taste. Furthermore, it alerts us when milk sours and food spoils. It is one of our 5 senses; smell, sight/vision, taste, hearing and touch which allows us to observe, process and integrate our reality.

The 5 senses can also be used to ingest, or perhaps the better expression is 'to immerse in', natural healing and remedies; 'food is medicine' (taste and digestion), music therapy (hearing), massage and manual therapy (touch), art therapy (vision), and yes, aromatherapy (smell). Mankind has been using aromatherapy and essential oils for millennia. The ancients recognized their healing effects on our constitution; from psychological states to physical ailments, as well as spiritual health (frankincense and myrrh to name a couple of biblical references). Essential oils provide us with a 'fragrant pharmacy'; organic, non-pharmacological, non-surgical relief from common, sub-clinical ailments with minimal side effects.

The use of aromatherapy was once considered fringe and anecdotal at best. But as the cost of medicine and health care continue to sky rocket, people are looking for ways to prevent these costly, but necessary services. "…Essential oils (are) now being used in general, maternity, and oncology hospital wards and in-care homes, and studied in research departments of universities. Aromatherapy has become a world-wide movement." - (The Complete Book of Essential Oils and Aromatherapy, Valerie Ann Worwood). I truly believe that natural, holistic, non-invasive therapies, such as those mentioned above, are powerful prevention and maintenance tools, especially when blended with the health pillars of whole food nutrition, restorative sleep and moderately stressful and varied physical activity.

As a massage therapist who has dabbled in aromatherapy and essential oils (EO's), I've come to learn that Lavender can have a calming and soothing effect that helps sedate the nervous system and facilitates sleep, Peppermint can have a stimulating effect that's also good for achy joints and sinus congestion. And Frankincense has a grounding effect that is great for clients riddled with anxiety and depression. Often, an EO can be used for a variety of symptoms and maladies. This would be analogous to the use of Wellbutrin or Cymbalta for both pain and depression.

I was slow to harness these benefits and incorporate essential oils in my private practice, but my enthusiasm for the art of aromatherapy was, and is, a direct reflection of the feedback I receive from my patients/clients. In fact, it wasn't until almost a full decade into my practice that I had my first exposure to essential oils…

If my memory serves, I was attending a massage convention; the yearly FSMTA (Florida State Massage Therapy Association) convention in 2005 in Boca Raton, Florida. Upon waking from my hotel slumber for the first day of classes, I struggled and suffered with a crick in my neck; a common ailment from sleeping in an unaccustomed bed. I wandered into the massage exhibit hall to peruse all the latest manual therapy books, tools and equipment. One of the first booths I walked by was an essential oil company's. The attendant noticed the pain and stiffness in my neck and beckoned me to her booth. She engaged me in small talk and inquired about my obvious neck discomfort. I explained what had occurred and I consented to an application of an EO blend for muscle pain and soreness. She then proceeded to rub the oil blend into my posterior neck and shoulder muscles for no longer than 30 seconds and requested I stop by her booth on the way out. I agreed and proceeded to wander through the massage exhibit hall maze over the next hour or so; catching up with colleagues, shopping for supplies and sampling different products. By the time I had completed my circuit through the hall, I had forgotten my promise to stop by the attendant's booth, but she caught my eye just as I approached the exit double doors. I sheepishly recognized my faux pas and approached her booth, as previously promised. We checked my neck movement and I was amazed at the almost complete resolution of my symptoms; both pain and stiffness were all but completely gone. Needless to say, I purchased the blend on the spot; my very first nudge into the greater world of essential oils.

Since then, I have attended several classes and researched several oils and blends, as well as various oil companies. I consider myself an aficionado rather than an adept, as I slowly added to my EO arsenal. I also use them in the shower as a form of natural body wash as well as a body cologne. Students who attend the massage school that I teach at, often share their stories and educate me on their own preferred EO's and blends. I know therapists that are completely immersed in the world of aromatherapy; including applications varying from infused massage oils, diffusers, bath bombs, natural remedies, inhalers, tinctures, etc.

As the EO industry continues to expand exponentially in popularity, the average newcomer struggles to find an essential resource that guides the neophyte into safe usage and the basics of essential oils and aromatherapy and its myriad applications. There are several books and quick references available. But how to decide? Do you want a quick reference or comprehensive tour of the fundamental concepts; history, verbiage, production, how to choose and store quality essential oils, tips, how they affect the body, mind and spirit, recipes, application, safety, and more?

Look no further than the book/pdf that you are now reading. In addition, the book is specifically written for manual and massage therapists. Written by an educator, producer and enthusiast of aromatherapy. It shows in the organization, depth and writing style. This is a book that is both accessible and also to be sipped, according to topic, like champagne. A book that you can come back to, again and again, to learn a different aspect of the art and science of aromatherapy. So, without further ado, I encourage you to start your journey, or perhaps, continue your journey down the sensual path of fragrances and healing.

Tedy Narvaez, LMT

16 March 2024

Preface

This book was created for massage therapists and bodyworkers to get real, personal, and informational tools to support the use of aromatherapy in their practices.

Beyond misting an aromatherapy blend on a pillow or linens.

Here, we are delving deep into the reasons why plants are powerful medicines, the cultivation and usage of essential oils, and how to assist our clients in having the most healing and holistic experience possible.

Do you want to learn more about how essential oils support the body, mind, spirit?

Do you want to uplevel your bodywork treatments?

Do you want to make your own aromatherapy based products?

This book is for you.

Let's go on a journey as old as time to unveil the healing of plants–and how to use essential oils, hydrosols, and herb oils in your own creative and intuitive way.

Table of Contents

Introduction

If you're a bodyworker–you've at least heard of aromatherapy. Maybe you use essential oils in your products for their analgesic, antispasmodic and relaxation properties. Maybe you take your clients on a sensory journey before your sessions, and use essential oils to help your clients relax.

Here, we're taking things a step further. My wish is for you to understand different plants and oils in such a way that you can create deeply transformative experiences for your clients.

Anxiety melting, nostalgia inducing, inflammation cooling, holistic HEALING.

I fell in love with aromatic botanicals at a young age. I remember hearing my dad talk about using herbal oils on my great grandmother for her back pain. I remember him rubbing arnica oil on my legs when they ached. I remember the relief. Growing up, we had a lot of experience working with our plant friends, and I am grateful for being introduced to herbal medicine at such a young age.

(Pictures of my dad and I harvesting and distilling hydrosol)

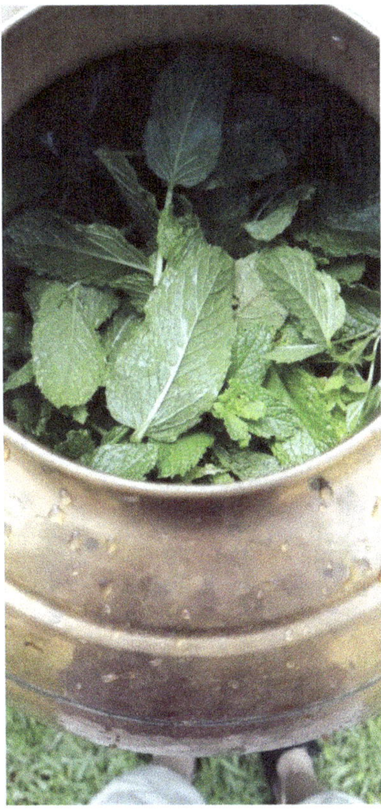
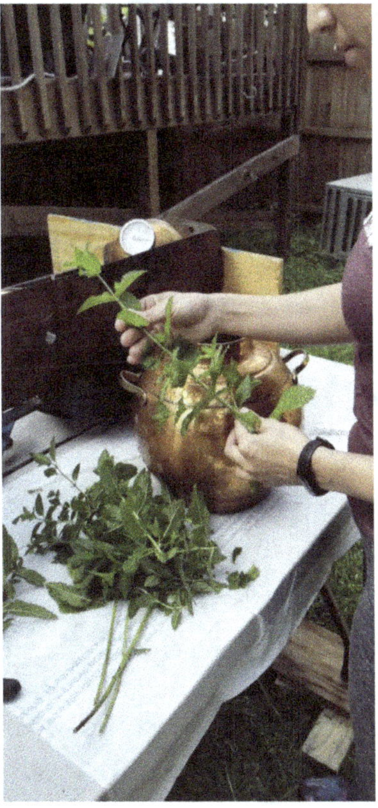

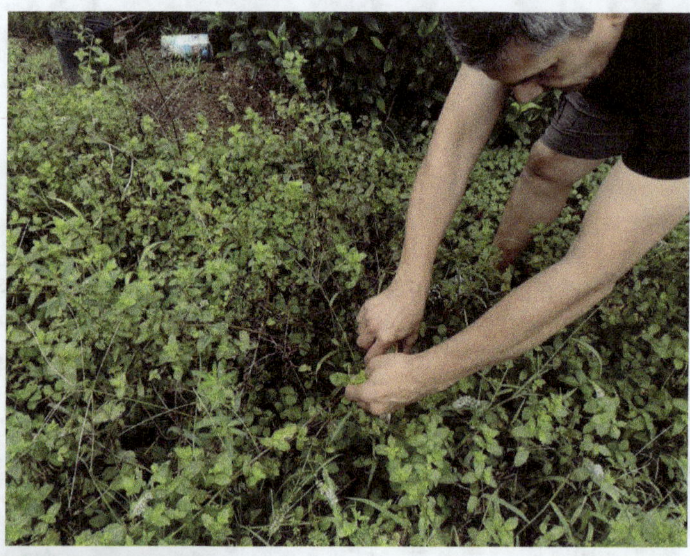

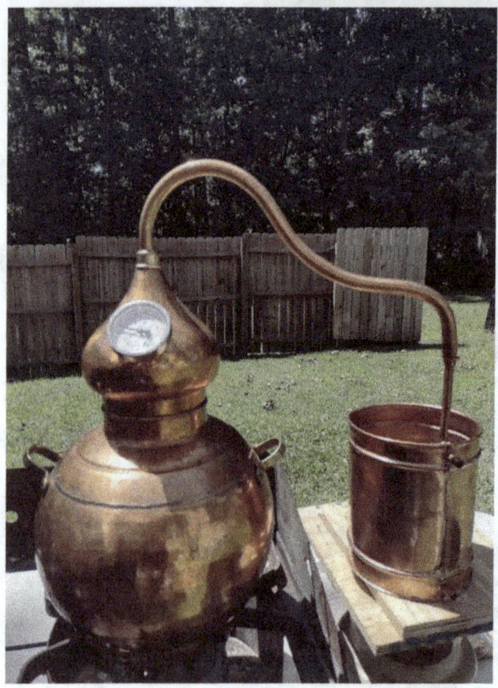

When I became a Massage Therapist at 19, I was excited to infuse my practice with my love for herbs, oils, and aromas. I knew this would enhance my treatments and enhance my client's experiences, and would fill up my cup, too.

Through the years, I've cultivated a really traditional and holistic approach to bodywork, and it's become something people come from all over the world to experience.

We get to make art here—we get to flavorize our treatments and let many modalities inspire our creative flow with clients. It's a beautiful dance, and one I want to empower more bodyworkers to try.

My mission is to give people a permission slip to take charge of their own health and wellbeing. Not to be a passive recipient of the healthcare system. We've got the power to create vitality from the inside out. We just need to get back to the basics.

When the body feels good, you just want to live in it!

I am excited to introduce to you a guide that you can refer to again and again along your journey with essential oils and aromatherapy.

This book provides a comprehensive overview of various essential oils and their therapeutic properties, practical techniques for incorporating aromatherapy into your bodywork practice, and plenty of amazing recipes for making your own massage oils, butter salves, and spa treatments.

How to Use this Book

Here, you'll find an abundance of information about holistic aromatherapy and its applications for bodyworkers. This book will serve as a foundation for you to implement aromatherapy into your own practice.

Each essential oil profile includes recipes for applying the oils therapeutically. Get as creative as you'd like with these! If you prefer to work with a butter as your base, you can substitute the massage oil and apply the essential oils used in the recipe to a massage butter. If you are newer to formulation -use the sample recipes until you get comfortable. And if you want to go crazy and swap out ingredients as you wish, go for it!

My only advice would be to stay within the framework for dilutions and the oils particular applications. Aromatherapy is NOT a one size fits all and not all oils are suitable for all applications, like in the bath or on the face.

Always get to know your oils before using them; not just the benefits but most importantly the safety precautions..

Now, before we dive in—I want to invite you to go grab your favorite essential oil—diffuse it or apply it (with a carrier oil) to your wrists and take five deep breaths…

"To reach the individual, we need an individual remedy. Each of us has a unique message. It is only the unique remedy that will suffice. We must, therefore, Cinco de Ferris substances which present affinities with the human being we intend to treat, those which will compensate for his deficiencies and those which will make his faculties blossom."

- Marguerite Maury, The Secret of Life and Youth

What is Aromatherapy?

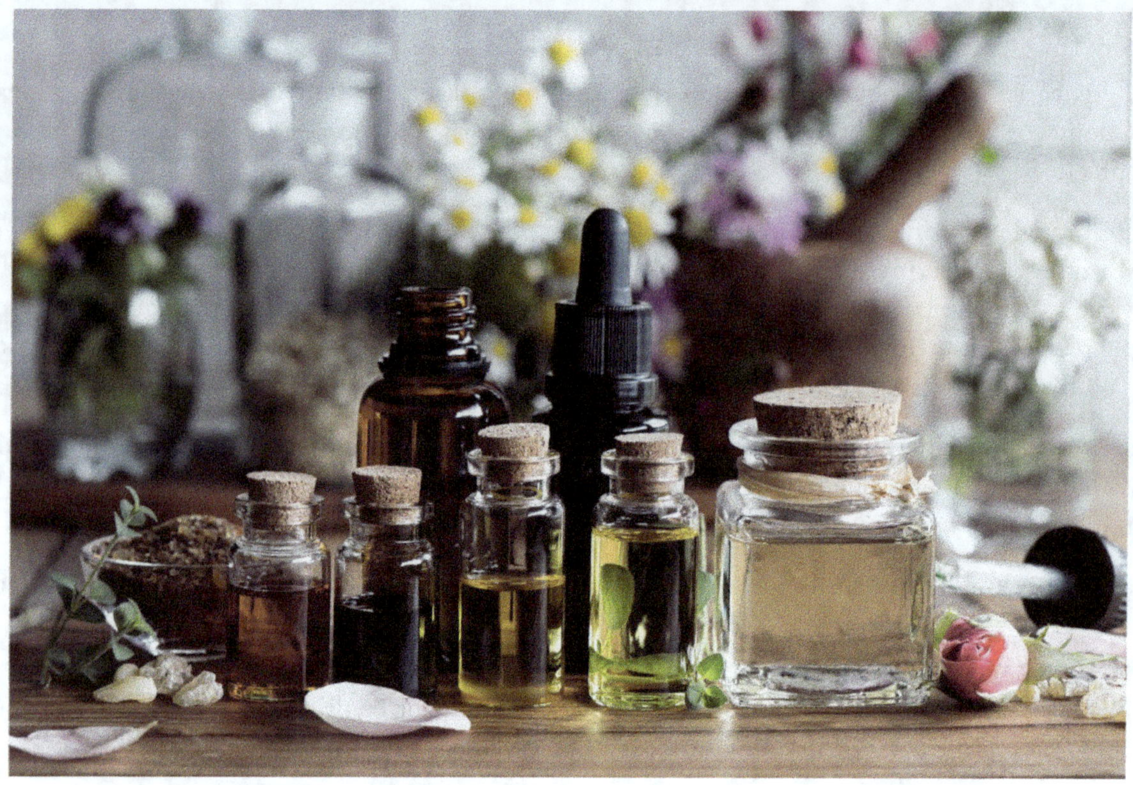

Aromatherapy – noun (aro·ma·ther·a·py) is the art and science of utilizing naturally extracted aromatic essences from plants to balance, harmonize, and promote wellness physically and psychologically. Plants are the source of oils, which contain the natural fragrances and therapeutic properties of the plant they come from. You can inhale, diffuse, apply diluted to the skin, or add them to a bath or wellness product.

We, as aromatherapists, believe that inhaling the scent of essential oils stimulates the brain to produce hormones and other neurochemicals that have a positive effect on the body.

Aroma: the aromatic substances that give essential oils their unique smell

Therapy: the therapeutic and healing nature of these plant essences

Together, the use of essential oils benefits both our physical and emotional wellbeing.

It is an art… when we tap into the creativity of formulation.

And it's a science because.. we study chemistry, anatomy, physiology, pathologies and plant constituents to work with essential oils.

Perhaps what I love most is that it's a holistic practice. It teaches us to look at the person as a whole, and we put the puzzle pieces together one by one—not solely focusing on symptoms, but rather the root of their dis-ease.

And we inspire them to take steps towards a happier and healthier life along the way.

> Take a moment to journal/ponder: In what ways can I be more of service to the whole with the tools I have available?

It's important to note that associations with smells are highly subjective and there are no set rules! What one finds pleasant, someone else will not.

When choosing your oils, make sure your client likes the aromas you're using—individually and in combination. If someone dislikes an aroma, it can lead to a strong, negative response. And in that state—it's almost impossible to relax.

Preferences can be affected by the season, the weather, and on's mood and emotional state. Just as our environment changes on a daily basis, so does the balance between our body and mind. That said, aromatics are wonderful allies through the changing seasons of our lives.

Aromatherapy falls under the category of Complementary and Alternative Medicine (CAM). Aromatherapy doesn't and shouldn't replace medical care. It can help amplify the benefits and/or outcomes of alternative medicines and wellness treatments; but it's only one slice of the big wellness pie, not an either-or sort of thing.

Merging the healing effects of aromatics with other therapies feeds the body, mind, and spirit. Aromatherapy helps soothe skin ailments, alleviates aches and pains, and helps restore an overtaxed nervous system. It can help open the heart, ground the spirit, and connect to ourselves.

When working optimally, our bodies intelligently know how to heal themselves. We strengthen that ability with modalities that keep us vital, strong, and enlivened on a cellular level.

Aromatherapy supports the body's healing process without weakening it. Rosemary helps with muscular tension and aching joints. It's also used for clearing and stimulating the mind, and relieving "brain fog" or mental fatigue. Learning about the healing properties of essential oils will empower you to enhance your therapeutic treatments, while using them safely and effectively with clients.

History on Plants as Medicine

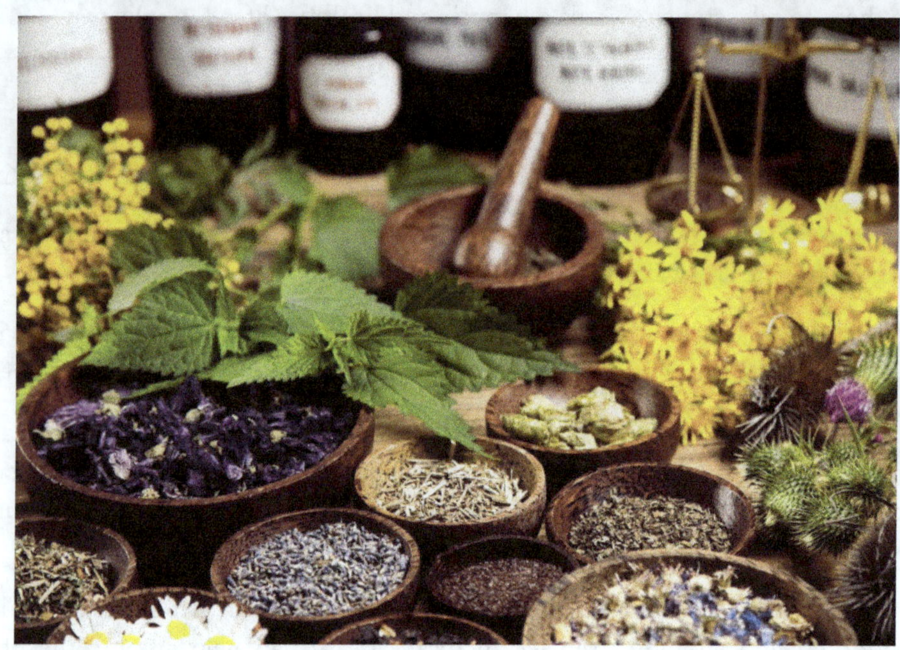

The art of using aromatic plants for well being is nothing new. Actually, it's older than mankind itself. Early ancient texts speak of different seeds and herbs being present at burial sites, and the making of oils, ointments, and salves with plants to heal the body.

It was trial and error at first, and because of the people who did the early work, we have an incredible amount of research to lean on about how plants heal and how to use them safely.

6,000 years ago, the Egyptians pioneered using scents and aromatics from plants to support the healing process. Then they passed their wisdom on to the Greeks and Romans—who were famous for their fine perfumes.

The Chinese, Indians, Greeks, and Romans used therapeutic oils to make perfumes, body care treatments, and medicines. People commonly used aromatic oils for spiritual, therapeutic, hygienic, and ritualistic purposes.

Ebers Papyrus

One text that got the party started—is Ebers Papyrus. EP is an ancient Egyptian medical text that dates back to around 1550 BC. It is one of the oldest medical texts in the world, and it contains a wealth of information on the medical practices and beliefs of the ancient Egyptians.

Georg Ebers, a German Egyptologist who discovered the papyrus in the 19th century, named it the Ebers Papyrus. The papyrus is written in the hieratic script, which the ancient Egyptians commonly used for religious texts and scientific texts.

The Ebers Papyrus divides into several sections, each addressing a different aspect of ancient Egyptian medicine. The papyrus covers a wide range of topics: surgery, obstetrics, pharmacology, nutrition, and more. It also includes detailed descriptions of physical ailments and treatments, and information on the use of herbs and natural remedies.

This historical document provides unique insight into the medical practices and beliefs of ancient Egyptians. It is also an important resource of the history of medicine, as it contains wisdom on the use of plants and other natural remedies in ancient medicine.

Pioneers of Aromatherapy

René-Maurice Gattefossé

In the early 20th century, a French chemist, René-Maurice Gattefossé, coined the term "aromatherapie" and was a powerful advocate of the use of essential oils for healing. Gattefossé discovered the healing properties of essential oils by accident when he burned his hand and plunged it into a vat of lavender oil, which helped to heal the wound and reduce scarring.

He then started analyzing the chemical properties of essential oils and how they treated burns, skin infections and wounds in soldiers during World War I. His book contains early clinical findings for utilizing essential oils for physiological ailments.

Gattefossé's intention using the word "Aromatherapie" meant that he wanted to distinguish the medicinal and therapeutic actions of essential oils from their perfumery applications.

Since then, aromatherapy has gained popularity as a complementary therapy for a variety of conditions like anxiety, stress, insomnia, and pain.

Dr Jean Valnet

Dr. Jean Valnet was a French physician and author who also helped pioneer modern aromatherapy. Valnet was a World War II veteran that became interested in the medicinal properties of essential oils after using them to treat soldiers who were suffering from physical and emotional ailments.

He studied the effects of essential oils on the human body and published several books, including "The Practice of Aromatherapy" and "Aromatherapy: The Treatment of Diseases by Plant Extracts."

Valnet's work played a crucial role in establishing aromatherapy as a legitimate form of alternative medicine, and his books continue to be regarded as important resources for those interested in the field. Valnet was also an advocate for environmental conservation and the use of natural remedies for health and wellness.

Marguerite Maury

Marguerite is a powerhouse in this field. She was a chemist, homeopath, aromatherapist and clinical researcher that made a massive imprint on how we understand essential oils and their benefits. She inspired the idea of taking a holistic approach with herbal products and to look at the whole body, mind, and spirit of the person.

Marguerite was born in Austria in 1906 and moved to France as a young woman. She became interested in natural beauty and began studying the essential oils for skin care and wellness.

> "Applied to the skin, these essences regulate the activity of the capillaries and restore vitality to the tissues. . . But of the greatest interest is the effect of (aroma) has on the psychic and mental state of the individual. Powers of perception become clearer and more acute. . . The use of odoriferous matter induces a true sentimental and mental liberation. . . the essential oils free us from the (a challenging emotion) but leave our faculties unimpaired."

Maury opened a beauty salon in Paris in the 1930s and developed a line of natural skin care products with essential oils. She wrote several books about aromatherapy and its uses in beauty treatments and health care. Maury's work helped make essential oils more popular in the beauty industry and she became a respected expert in aromatherapy.

She believed in taking a holistic and unique approach with each person, realizing this is not a one size fits all solution; and she brought light to the mental benefits of working with herbal oils.

Robert Tisserand

Robert is a well-known expert in essential oils and aromatherapy. He travels internationally to educate people about the safe and effective use of essential oils in medicine.

Robert Tisserand, is the man.

He established one of the first companies in Britain to sell essential oils to the public, and co-founded the Tisserand Institute—an organization that provides education and training on getting the most out of using essential oils, in the safest way possible.

He also wrote many of "the books" on aromatherapy. I recommend them all.

> The Art of Aromatherapy
> The Essential Oil Safety Handbook
> Essential Oil Safety: A Guide for Health Care Professionals

Jeffrey Yuen

Jeffrey Yuen is a renowned practitioner and teacher of Chinese Medicine that has made significant contributions to the field of aromatherapy. He's known for integrating the use of essential oils with acupuncture, herbal medicine, and Qi Gong.

According to Yuen, aromatherapy plays a significant role in meeting the requirements of all three preconditions of life: Survival (access to nutrition and the ability to fill fundamental physiological needs), Interaction (specifically interactions with other humans) and Differentiation (the ability to adopt or refine our habits as we go through life).

He also has a really beautiful perspective on the energetics of essential oils. According to Chinese Medicine, every substance, including plants and their essences, has specific properties that affect the body's Qi or life force. Yuen has identified the therapeutic properties of essential oils and their correspondences with the various organs, meridians, and elements in Chinese Medicine.

His use of essential oils with acupuncture or acupressure led him to develop specific protocols for working with essential oils (topically or by inhalation) during sessions. He believes that incorporating aromatherapy enhances both the immediate and longer-term benefits of the session. Chinese medicine always aims to remedy the imbalance rather than counteracting the symptoms.

Aromatherapy Today

Since Gattefossé's time, aromatherapy has been used to treat a wide range of physical and emotional conditions–including stress, anxiety, depression, insomnia, and chronic pain. It has been used to support the immune system, improve digestion, and promote overall physical and emotional well-being. We saw the beginnings of modern Aromatherapy in France, then in England–where they began integrating aromatherapy with hands on touch and massage.

And like wildfire, it spread throughout the world.

When that fire came to the US, it was in the form of toiletries and "smell good" gifts, not in therapy. This gave it a bad rap, because low-quality oils were being used and there was little focus on quality or therapeutic benefits.

Adulterated oils were being sold as pure, and it created an uphill battle for aromatherapists. But we've come a long way in the states and now there are more professionals and educated consumers prioritizing high quality oils for their therapeutic applications.

This is a main reason we continue to have the conversation of the value of *genuine* aromatherapy and how to source high quality, high potency essential oils.

Side Note: Fragrance oils are frowned upon by holistic aromatherapists. They are synthetic chemicals used in common toiletries but lack therapeutic value. When we refer to Aromatherapy, we are referring to the distilled or expressed *natural plant essence called an Essential Oil.*

Our Role as Bodyworkers

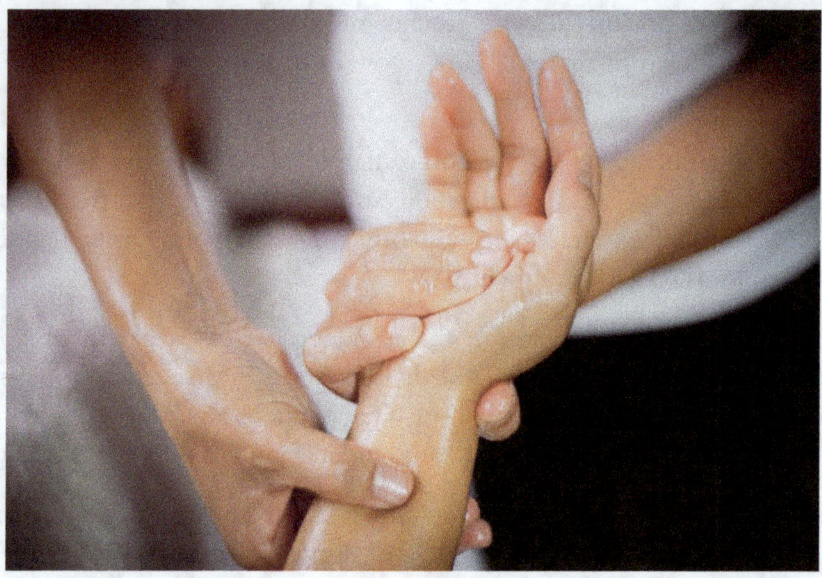

"It is compassion, then, that is the best protection; it is also, as the great masters of the past have always known, the source of all healing."

Sogyal Rinpoche

In the world of massage and bodywork, we've still got plenty of work to do. Most commercial spas offer only a handful of essential oils for aromatherapy use—usually lavender, eucalyptus, and a couple others. They may add an essential oil to their massage medium or diffuse an oil in the room—but it's far from a holistic approach.

So what exactly do we mean by holistic aromatherapy and how can it support our practice?

Holistic aromatherapy involves using pure, high-quality oils matched with a comprehensive view of the person. It means choosing oils that will support specific ailments and organ systems and using them in a variety of ways to enhance the healing process.

Plant essences are allies and the more we get to know and work with them, the better we can support our clients. Massage therapists create a multisensory experience that is highly individualized. We all have different needs at different times, and we show up a little differently every day.

How many times have you dropped in with a client to see how they are feeling…*today?* It can be a drastic change from the time you last saw them. It's crucial for this healing journey with our clients to continue to have open dialogue and to ask questions so you can meet them where they are.

Your sessions will drastically enhance as you become more and more confident with the knowledge of plant essences and how they work with the body.

What Are Essential Oils?

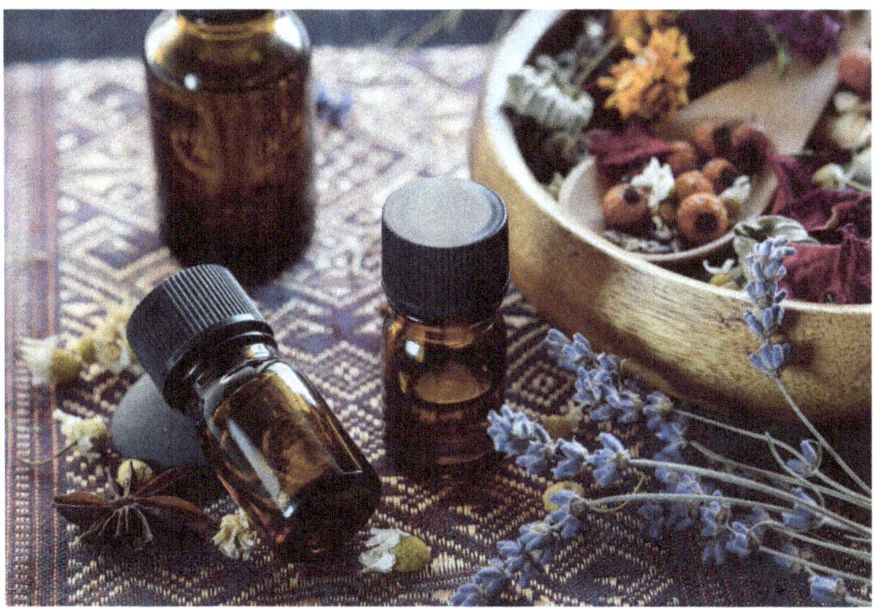

"Perhaps it was the flowers that made me a painter." - Monet

Essential oils capture the very essence of nature.

They are the concentrated extracts derived from different parts of a plant including: the roots, leaves, seeds, resins, barks and flowers. Some plants produce more than one kind of essential oil. The bitter orange tree produces orange from the rind of the fruit, Petitgrain from the leaves, and Neroli from the blossoms.

Fun fact: It can take approximately a pound of peppermint leaves to make a drop of Peppermint Essential Oil and approximately 50 rose flowers to create a single drop of Rose Oil!

Some plants produce very little Essential Oil, however, produce an abundance of beautiful hydrosol (which we'll get to later)!

You should never underestimate these highly concentrated precious oils. Even when used sparingly, they offer immense therapeutic benefit. Less is always more. Some plants yield more essential oil than others; which is one reason pricing ranges can be across the board.

It's important to note that essential oils are NOT fragrance or perfume oils! Lab-made perfume oils containing artificial chemicals do not provide the therapeutic benefits that essential oils offer.

Using undiluted essential oils topically is rare. An exception would be to place a drop of lavender on a bug bite to relieve inflammation and itching or tea tree oil on a scratch.

Essential oils are also not oily like vegetable oils. Most are transparent or have various hues, such as yellow (Turmeric), orange (Sweet Orange) and blue (Australian Blue Cypress).

They are:

    A). Lipophilic - soluble in oil
    B). Hydrophobic - not soluble in water
    C). They are volatile, evaporate like alcohol, and some are flammable.

The complex chemical composition of Essential Oils, also known as constituents, is how we receive the therapeutic benefits through inhalation and/or external application.

You should always know about an essential oil before using it on yourself or another person. This reduces the likelihood of an adverse reaction.

Why do Plants produce Essential Oils?

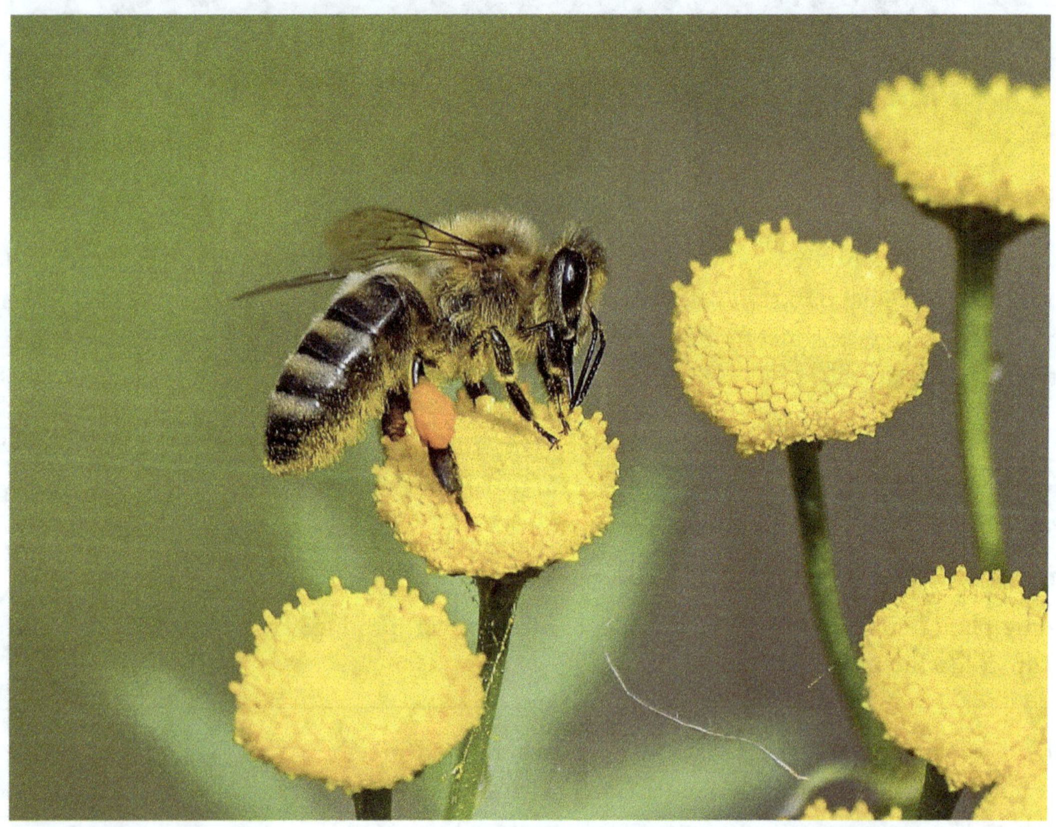

The short answer–for many of the same reasons we use them. To heal, to protect, and to keep themselves vital and thriving.

Plants produce Essential Oils for:

Protection- Antimicrobial, anti-fungal and anti-bacterial properties have been well documented. The Aquilaria tree, among other plants known to man, releases a healing resin formed in the heartwood (agarwood) when it experiences a wound or fungal infection.

Defense- To defend itself against insects or other animals. Some essential oils contain insect repelling properties, while other plants can be displeasing by causing nausea or being toxic to mammals when eaten.

To attract pollinators- We are not the only ones who enjoy the fragrance of flowers. Other species do as well!

Allelopathy- Yes, plants compete and suppress other plants! This occurs when a plant releases biochemicals (known as allelochemicals) to prevent other vegetation from growing within its zone.

Where are the essential oils stored in the plants?

Essential Oils are found wherever the plant's secretory structures are.

Here are some examples:

A). Rose (Rosaceae): flower petals
B). Eucalyptus & Tea Tree: oil sacs
C). Peppermint & Clary Sage: glands on surface of leaves
D). Yarrow: entire plant
E). Vetiver & Ginger: roots
F). Juniper & Carrot Seed: berries and seeds
G). Orange Tree: blossoms, rind of fruit, leaves
H). Cedarwood, Ho Wood, & other barks
I). Frankincense, Copaiba and Myrrh: resins

The flower petals of a Rose (Rosaceae) contain them, as well as the oil sacs in the leaves of the eucalyptus and tea tree (Myrtaceae family), and the glands on the surface of leaves like peppermint and clary sage (Labiatae).

Some plants undergo distillation of the entire herb, such as Yarrow (Composite), while others utilize the flowering tops including the petals, stalks, and leaves, like Lavender.

Essential Oils are also extracted from roots (Vetiver and Ginger), and berries & seeds (Juniper and Carrot Seed). The orange tree produces aromatic oil from its blossoms, the rind of the fruit and the leaves. Cedarwood, Ho wood, and other barks are extracted for their essence while Frankincense, Copaiba and Myrrh the oil are extracted from their resins.

How Are Essential Oils Extracted?

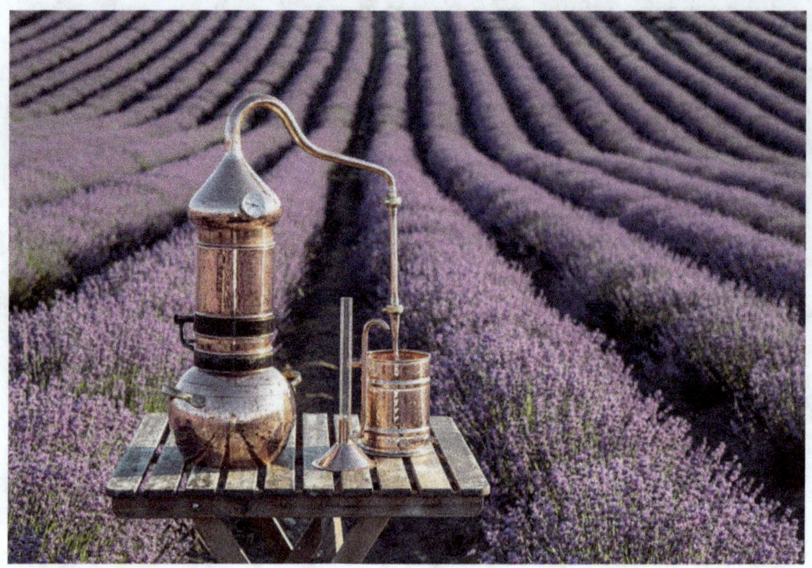

Essential Oil distillers typically extract Essential Oils by one of the two methods below, and they isolate a true essential oil by physical means only. Since essential oils extract the volatile molecules of the plant, that's where the essence is.

Steam Distillation

Steam Distillation is the most common and widely known process of extracting essential oils. In this method, essential oils are physically separated from the water phase.

The distillation process begins with compact storing the harvested plant in a large steel or copper vessel, so there is no room for air pockets.

Fewer air pockets= more oil

Once the vessel is fully filled, it is closed tightly and exposed to an oil-fired boiler. The boiler heats water into steam, which is then injected into the bottom of the still at shallow pressure.

Then the steam gradually rises to the top of the still heating the plant inside as it moves to the top. The steam bursts the glands in the plant's composition, releasing its fragrant oil. At the same time, cold water is channeled within the vessel to condense the steam containing the oil.

This water and oil mixture is then left to set, allowing separate layers to form. The oil is then removed from the water and processed for use.

Expression (cold press)

Citrus oils are commonly produced by the method of cold pressing. Oils like lemon, bergamot, mandarin, grapefruit, orange and lime are all extracted by this method.

> Fun Fact: Citrus fruits are extremely rich and essential oils. In the past, people used to do this process by hand, but today machines are used.

Using an orange as our example, the device mechanically pierces the whole fruit to rupture the essential oil sacs, which are located on the underside of the rind. The oils run down into a collection receptacle. Then, the whole fruit is pressed to squeeze out the juice and the oil.

The oil and juice that are produced still contain solids from the fruits, such as the peel, and must be centrifuged to filter the solids from the liquids. The oil separates from the juice layer and is siphoned off into another receptacle.

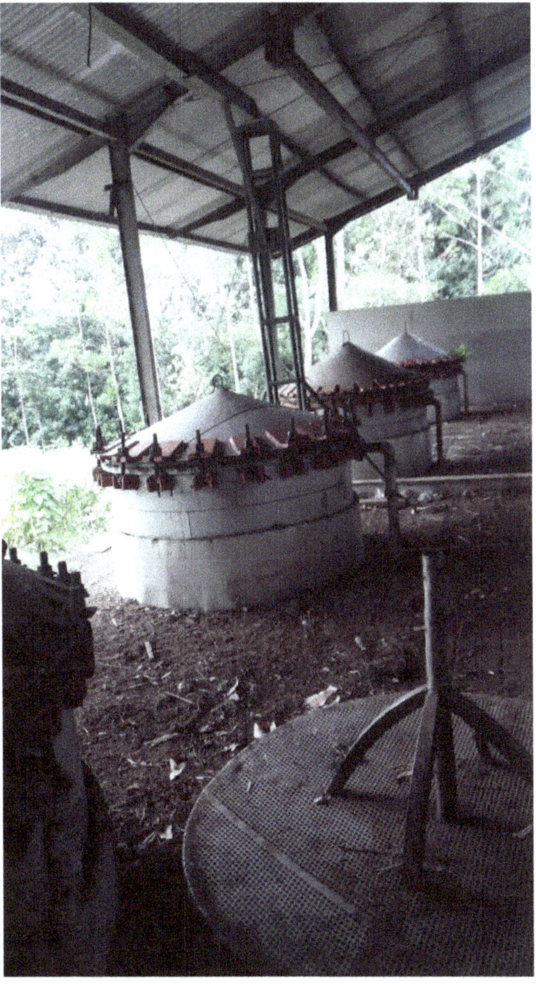

(Farm Distillation from Wild Harvest Indonesia)

Other Aromatics

While the following are not essential oils, they have immense therapeutic value and are often used by aromatherapists:

Absolutes

Absolutes are aromatic substances that are obtained by enfleurage or solvent extraction. This method is used when we're dealing with delicate flowers that are too fragile to be distilled using heat or pressure. To extract the volatile elements, the petals are soaked in a spirit solvent and then evaporate the solvent with alcohol to separate the aromatic compounds from the pigments and waxes.

We're left with the beautiful and odoriferous material from the plant—and we call this an absolute.

The fragrances of absolutes are richer and thicker in consistency than those of distilled or cold pressed essential oils, so they may need to be warmed to be malleable.

We get the absolutes from flowers like jasmine, lotus, gardenia, violet leaf, and tuberose using this process.

CO2 Extracts

The CO2 (carbon dioxide) method extracts aromatics that are referred to as CO2 Extracts.

CO2 extraction involves passing carbon dioxide through plant material at a high enough pressure that it becomes "supercritical." Supercritical carbon dioxide is in a sweet spot where it moves into a physical state, rather than acting as a gas or a liquid. Then it can be used as a solvent to extract aromatic oils from certain plants.

> Fun Fact: This method is extremely environmentally friendly and the constituents we are able to collect are incredibly stable and have a longer shelf life than most aromatics!

The resins of frankincense and myrrh, the roots of ginger, and the petals of roses are all viable for this method.

The composition of CO2 extracts are different from the equivalent essential oil—so they will have slightly different therapeutic characteristics. CO2 creates more medicinally active base oils, like we see with sea buckthorn and evening primrose.

Enfleurage

Enfleurage is one of the original methods for extracting essential oils, and the result is extraordinary! Pioneered back in the 18th century in France–this ancient art works simply and organically. Various producers of essential oils still use this method.

The principle: Fats dissolve essential oils and thereby absorb their aromas.

In the early days, it was common practice to soak lard or tallow with delicate flowers and flower petals to absorb their aromas over the series of several days. They would remove the old flowers, add new ones, and continue this cycle for a period of time until the fat was fully saturated. Then–the fat was dissolved by alcohol, the alcohol evaporated, and you were left with only the beautiful fragrance from the plant.

The catch is, you have to use a massive amount of plant material and the process is very labor intensive. In one study, 1000 kilos of tuberose blossoms yielded only 801 grams of oil. So this makes these oils very rare, very potent, and a bit hard to find.

Hydrosols – Healing Aromatic Waters

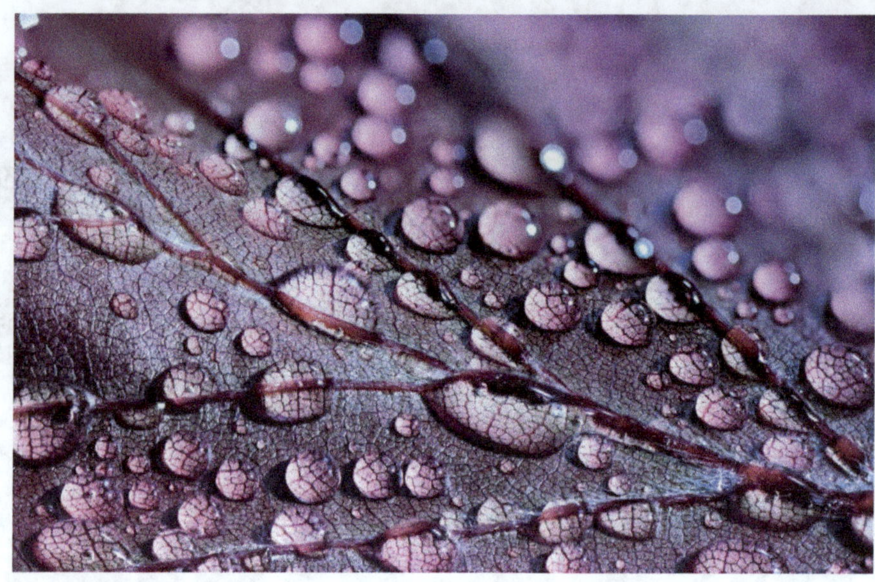

I absolutely love the conversation around hydrosols, because we don't talk about them enough.

Hydrosols are the healing aromatic waters produced as a product of distillation. They can be collected from the same distillation process used for essential oils, though sometimes distillation is used specifically for hydrosols.

Did you know that hydrosols have been used since ancient times, even before essential oils, by the Egyptians, Greeks, and Romans? They simply soaked the plant material in boiling water to absorb their healing properties. They used the water for health and beauty products to help heal wounds and to soothe the soul.

This aromatic water contains all of the water soluble constituents of the plant, some of which are not found in essential oils. Remember, essential oils are oil soluble, so they only contain those particular constituents.

Many people don't know that distillation isn't just for essential oils, it's for these beautiful healing waters as well! It takes so much plant material to extract the tiniest amount of oil, which is why pure essential oils can be so expensive. Using the hydrosols from distillation is a price effective alternative, and is safe for vulnerable groups like children, the elderly, and those who may be concerned about the potency of essential oils.

BEWARE OF THE TERM FLORAL WATERS!

There are many products sold on the market with the name floral water. Some of these contain drops of synthetic fragrance or maybe essential oil in water. This is not a true hydrosol. The definition of a true hydrosol is one that is extracted through the distillation of the plant.

Hydrosol Applications:

Facial Toners

Apply short bursts of hydrosol to rehydrate your skin, and for a quick refresh anytime of day.

Compress

Hydrosols can be used to make botanical compresses. By taking a clean cloth and damping it in a hydrosol, you can then apply that to an affected area of your body. This brings comfort to sore muscles, cramps, insect bites, and rashes.

Bath

The water of hydrosol is perfect for a rejuvenating bath. All you need is 1-2 cups of hydrosol mixed in your water. Enjoy!

Footbaths

Hydrosols really amp up footbaths. Peppermint and Rosemary are my favorite.

Neti Pot

When rinsing your sinuses using a neti pot, try adding 1 tsp of hydrosol water to have a better impact in tackling nasal congestion.

Laundry

Hydrosols can also be used to freshen your laundry. Some great hydrosol solutions for laundry cleaning are Lime (Citrus aurantifolia), Orange (Citrus sinensis), Lavender (Lavandula angustifolia), and Rose Geranium (Pelargonium Roseum). Toss your clothes in prepared hydrosol water, followed by drying them in a dryer. This freshens the cloth fibers and adds an aromatic element to your clothes!

Spritz

Spray hydrosols throughout your spaces for a revitalizing aroma!

In the Kitchen

Since hydrosols are naturally obtained, they can be used in the kitchen too! Try spraying Basil (Ocimum basilicum), Sage (Salvia sclarea), and Rosemary (Rosmarinus officinalis) hydrosols when roasting chicken or boiling pasta.

Essential Oil Quality & Tips When Purchasing

With so many "essential oils" on the market, it's important to know what to look for so you can source high quality oils that are safe and free from adulteration. The FDA doesn't regulate the purity or quality of essential oils, so you'll have to be your own advocate when shopping around.

Purchase From Reputable Suppliers

When sourcing aromatics and botanicals, find your local artisans and herbalists! Shopping locally is a beautiful thing and helps support your community in amazing ways; and besides that–this is where you are going to find the most ethically sourced and high-quality oils in your area.

While you may not find *every* ingredient you need, you should be able to find many wonderful, locally sourced raw ingredients to work into your products and services.

The Look & The Label

Essential oils should be light, non-greasy, and mostly clear. Companies that produce high quality essential oils package their products in dark amber glass bottles or PET plastic, which is non-toxic and 100% recyclable. The bottle should also have an orifice reducer to reduce oxygen degradation.

On the label–be sure to look for proper botanical names and the chemotypes of each plant, and be aware of the country of origin and the part of the plant being used.

Treat essential oils as medicine- storing in a cool, dark place and keeping away from children.

Adulterations

Oftentimes for the sake of profit–unethical producers will add things like alcohol, cheaper essential oils, and/or synthetic chemicals into their products.

For example–we know that rose oil, which is costly to produce, can sometimes be adulterated with oils like geranium essential oil, which is less costly. Lemon balm produces very little oil through distillation, so sometimes other plants are added to the distillation process to dilute them.

Lavandin can be labeled and sold as lavender, and the list goes on. This is why it is so important to become informed and to purchase from a reputable supplier!

GC/MS

There are two tests used in the world of essential oils that help to identify potential adulterations–the Gas Chromatography and Mass Spectrometry tests.

These "identity tests" report what chemical constituents are in each oil and the oil's chemical makeup. The resulting "fingerprint" or report allows for an experienced chemist to positively verify the oils identity. For each batch of oil, a reputable supplier *should* produce a GC/MS Certificate of Analysis that is current.

Soil conditions, elevation, weather, cultivation and harvesting methods, and the plant's environment all contribute to the constituents of the essential oil. Experts recommend having oils analyzed by a lab that specializes specifically in essential oil analysis because interpreting these tests depends highly on the skill, experience, and knowledge of the chemist.

To recap, a quality essential oil is:

- Grown in its indigenous area
- Harvested at peak time
- Properly distilled
- Free from adulterations or additives

How Essential Oils Work on the Body & Mind

Now that we've covered the framework of what aromatherapy and essential oils are, their origin story, the process of extraction, and how to make quality purchases... let's explore how these oils affect the body, mind, and spirit.

The pathway of Olfaction to our Limbic System

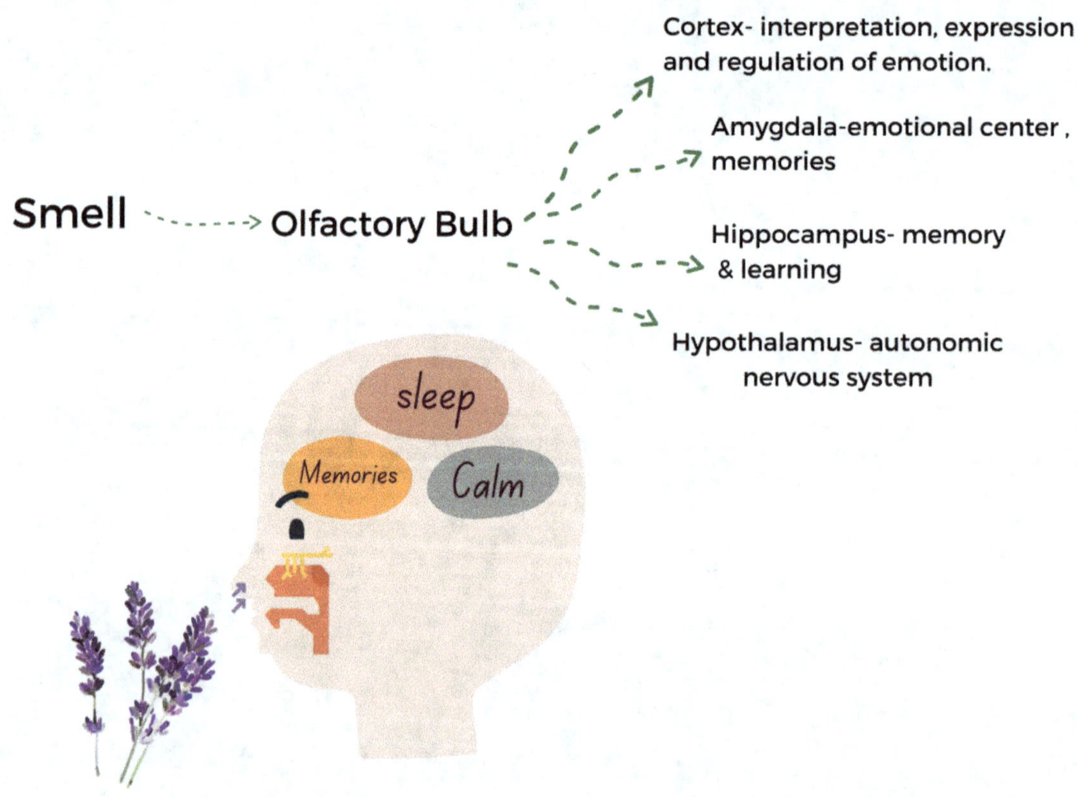

The Nervous System...where it all takes place

The Mind

When we inhale, diffuse, or use essential oils in a wellness product–what is actually giving us that vivid therapeutic and psychological benefit?

In short, when the scent molecules enter our nose, they travel through our olfactory nerves and directly into the brain–specifically affecting our brain's limbic system and emotional center. The term "emotion" is derived from the Latin "movere"–which means to move. Perhaps this is why we say we are "moved" when feeling an intense emotion.

Essential oils inspire us by elevating our sensory impressions with their distinct fragrance- the breath of the living plant. Aromatics influence us subtly by enhancing our awareness in a similar way that observing a painting or listening to music does.

You can also think of your emotions as energy-in-motion. Emotions are our way of relating to the world around us and attaching meaning to experiences in our life. We can experience them both consciously and subconsciously.

The Limbic System, also known as the emotional brain, is responsible for emotional feelings, our circadian rhythms, sleep and waking cycles, memories, motivational drives, and learning.

The Limbic System houses the hypothalamus, amygdala, and hippocampus.

We know that aromatics have a direct effect on these physiological changes because of their direct impact on the amygdala and hypothalamus. Therefore, aromatherapy continues to come forth as one of the most rapid and non-toxic ways to elevate the mood and still the mind.

Hypothalamus

Think of the hypothalamus like our built it stabilizer. Its job is to keep us in a state of homeostasis– and it does so by regulating our hormones and making subtle changes based on our internal and external environmental cues.

The hypothalamus responds to things like body temperature, hunger, thirst, blood pressure levels, hormone levels, cortisol expression, and our circadian rhythm–and brings us back into balance by working in conjunction with our endocrine and nervous systems.

Amygdala

The amygdala is our integrative center for emotions, emotional behavior, and motivation. It consists of two almond-shaped clusters of nuclei that rest in each temporal lobe of the brain. At the start: By initiating our "fight or flight" response, it plays a significant role in our response to fear and has a significant influence on our autonomic nervous system. It also controls various autonomic functions, such as respiration and regulating heart rhythm.

The amygdala helps us attach emotional meaning to our memories, helps us with decision making, and our reward center. It houses the main circuits that color our experience with emotion. It is also very responsive to aromas, which influences the autonomic nervous system.

Hippocampus

Located deep in the temporal lobe of the brain—the hippocampus plays a key role in our learning and memory imprinting. It is important in helping us retain longer term memories and regulates much of our emotional response. This intricate brain structure is very fragile and is easily damaged by different stimuli.

We see a decline in the size and function of the hippocampus with untreated severe depression, the onset of Alzheimer's, and lack of physical activity.

Longer Pathway for other senses

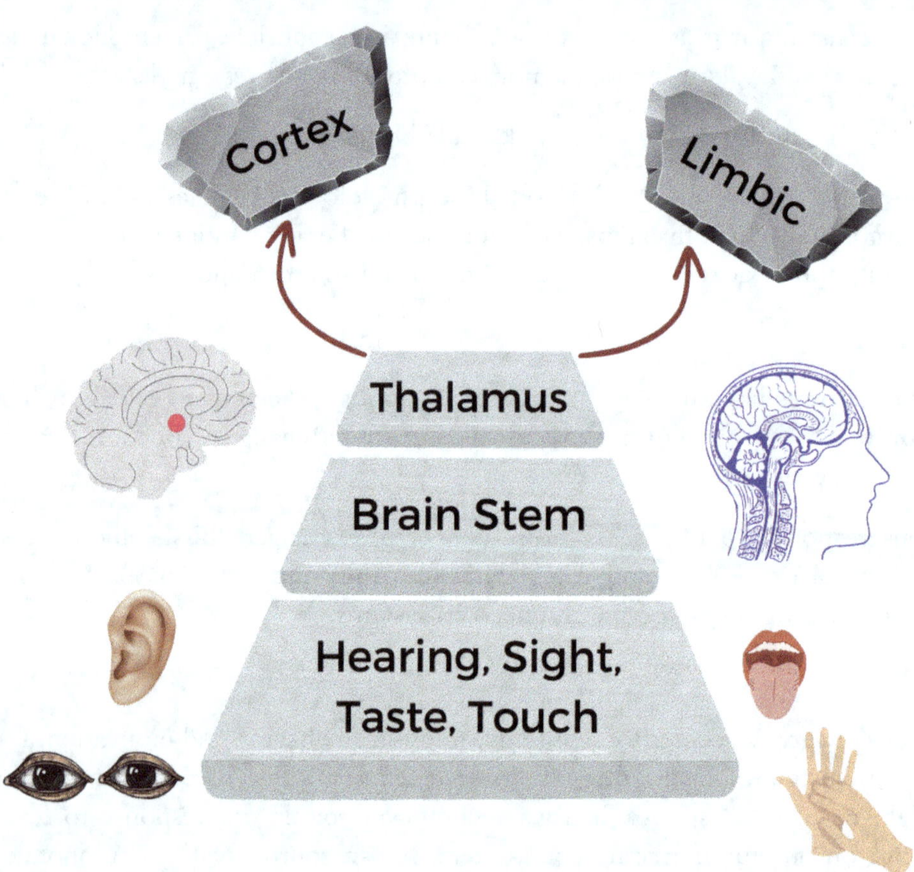

Supporting the Nervous System

As aromatherapists, our goal is to help regulate the nervous system's stress response. That said, oftentimes we cannot take people out of their environment or situations, especially those with PTSD and other mental health issues.

So how can we be of service? We can help support the nervous system and how it responds.

We simply cannot dab on some lavender and expect our problems to go away. However, we can work to find a place that makes us feel centered with the aid of aromatics. Porges' polyvagal (PLV) theory states that when we are "feeling connected," our ventral vagal system is in charge.

Our ventral vagal system is primarily responsible for promoting social engagement and interpersonal connection. It contributes to our emotional resilience and flexibility; and when active and healthy–makes us feel relaxed and safe.

The Properties of Plants

Working with Aromatics means working directly with the plant kingdom. One thing I hear all the time: "How can an oil have so many properties and benefits, often seeming contradictory?"

The versatility and complexity of nature is amazing, and we are continuing to uncover hidden secrets and uses of plant extracts all the time. It's hard not to be completely in awe of nature's complexity and the countless possibilities that lie within each herb.

Our relationship with Aromatics is as multifaceted as our relationship with other humans. Each plant contains a multitude of different constituents that together create a complete aroma.

How do we get to know these complex creations? By working with them over a long period of time; by practicing (creating formulations), reading books (studying about them), and, most importantly, using them with ourselves.

Aromatic Imprinting

Have you ever taken a whiff of a particular fragrance and felt transported to a time when you were young hanging out at grandma's house? This is called aromatic imprinting– and it happens when we attach a particular aroma to a memory.

Plant essences have the power to generate changes in the mind by connecting a scent and a memory emotion together. When we take in an aroma–nerve impulses reach the limbic system and activate smell related emotions and behaviors.

For example, the smell of orange essential oil might remind you of a warm summer afternoon when someone was peeling an orange on the porch. The smell of spruce essential oil might remind you of your trip in the Mountains breathing the crisp, fresh air. Each essential oil has unique chemical properties that affect us in a variety of ways, whether it's: relaxing, stimulating, pain relieving, warming, cooling, mentally clarifying, sedating, or grounding.

For me, lemongrass brings me back to Thailand. It grows like wildfire there and it's used often in their cuisine and herbal therapies.

We need to be aware that each person's experience with aromas will vary and will affect each person differently. What might bring back a warm summer camp trip for someone could bring back the day they lost their pet in the woods to another. Communicating with our clients to discover which aromas are pleasant to them is so important, and it helps us learn which aromas we may not want to use.

General rule of thumb—don't use a scent that isn't pleasant to you. That's an indicator that it won't work for you in the best way. I like to say "the nose knows". Our intuition knows best here.

Aromas have the power to instantly awaken memories or experiences of the past. Every person has a series of unique experiences, and aromatherapy can bring back life to those past experiences as if it was yesterday. The link between aromas and emotions goes much deeper than just a sense of smell. The powerful impact that scents can have on your mind is because of how they weave directly within the brain's limbic system, which houses our bank of emotions and other vital functions like memory creation and metabolism regulation.

Have you ever heard someone say they're not really hungry, but as soon as someone starts cooking within proximity, they get the tummy rumbles?

Aromas can stimulate the beginning of the digestive process and we even begin to physically salivate when we're near delicious food.

In a more primal sense, smell also serves as a defense mechanism for protection. We can smell and sense danger, which stimulates our fight-or-flight response to keep us alive. How do we know a fire must be near? We smell smoke.

Research Effects of Aromas

Over the years, scientists have studied and researched aromas and essential oils to explore their effect on our physiological responses and how they can provide support for conditions like stress, anxiety, depression, pain, and inflammation.

Since the inhalation of essential oils communicates directly with our olfactory system and stimulates the brain to release neurotransmitters like serotonin and dopamine—aromas serve as brilliant mood and sleep cycle regulators, and help us with alertness and concentration.

Let's check out a few examples:

Ylang Ylang is indicated for depression, anxiety, hypertension, frigidity, stress and palpitations (T. Hongratanaworakit, G. Buchbauer Relaxing effect of ylang ylang oil on humans after transdermal absorption,Phytother Res, 20 (2006)

One constituent in Lavender essential oil, Linalool, shows effectiveness for patients with sleep disturbance patterns, improving the feeling of wellbeing, supporting mental alertness and suppressing aggression and anxiety [P.H. Koulivand, M.K. Ghadiri, A. Gorji)

Oils high in 1,8 cineole (such as Rosemary, Eucalyptus and Bay Laurel) increased cerebral blood flow in humans after inhalation in a study. These oils are known to increase mental clarity and cognitive performance. Effects of 1,8-Cineole and (–)-Linalool on Functional Brain Activation in a Working Memory Task, Flavor and Fragrance Journal, May 2018

Aromatherapy and Anxiety: Aromatherapy, including the use of bergamot essential oil, has been studied for its effects on anxiety. A 2015 study published in the Journal of Alternative and Complementary Medicine found that inhaling bergamot essential oil vapor reduced anxiety levels and improved mood in patients awaiting minor surgery.

Limbic Response and Holding Space

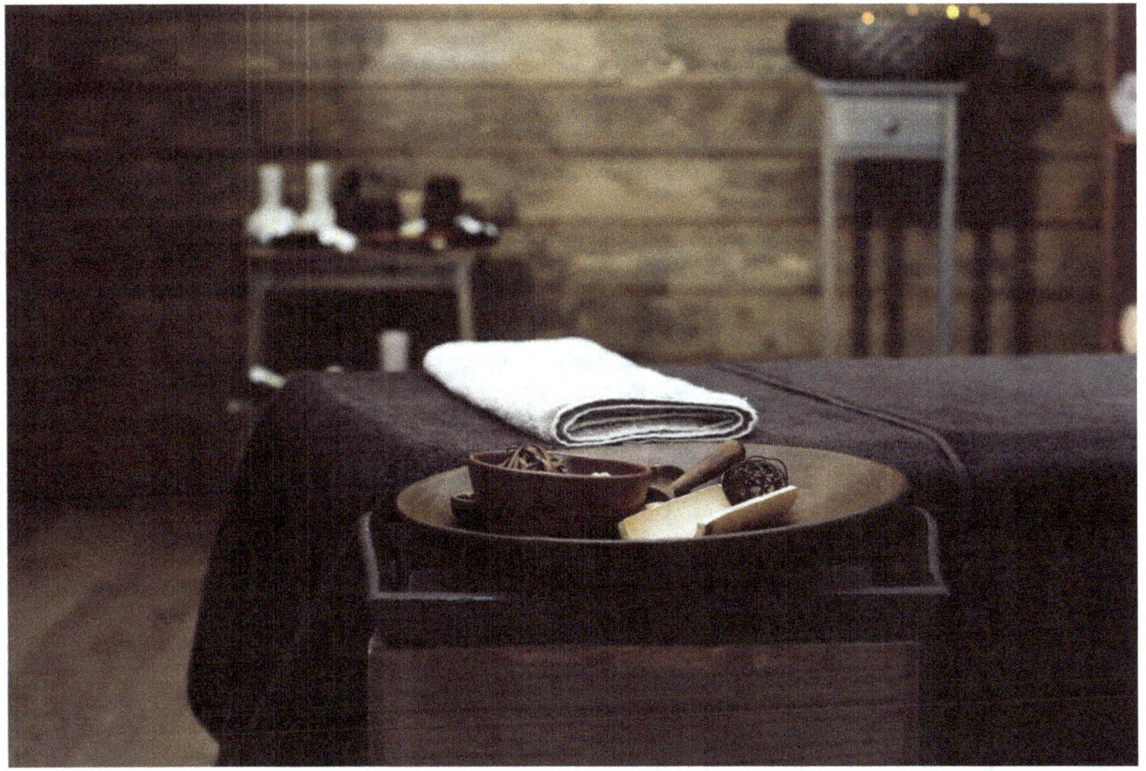

One of the key roles we play as bodyworkers is holding space for our clients. Holding a container for them to feel, to relax, and to connect to their true essence. As you well know, all sorts of things can come up during a bodywork session- and it's important to pay close attention so that you can give your clients the most supportive experience possible.

When we learn to use holistic aromatherapy to its fullest within our treatments–the space we hold becomes so much more enjoyable and soothing for our clients. It becomes a place where they can feel safe to resurface older memories and to create new ones.

I can't tell you how rewarding it is when a scent activates one of my clients' limbic response and they share their stories with me. I remember a session years ago when the scent of spruce oil took my client back to hiking in Canada. He told me how his friend cut himself with a hatchet and he used the sap of a conifer tree and applied it to the wound.

On the other side of the coin–keep in mind the memories that surface can be positive or negative. Always listen to the verbal cues from your clients, and ask good questions! Tune in with them to see if there are any aromas they are adverse to; and go from there.

Healing doesn't just take place in the treatment room, it continues long after they've left your table. We can support this continuously healing experience by offering gentle suggestions for self care (within your scope and training of course), and by empowering them to take ownership of their own health and vitality.

Traditional Chinese Medicine and Ayurveda

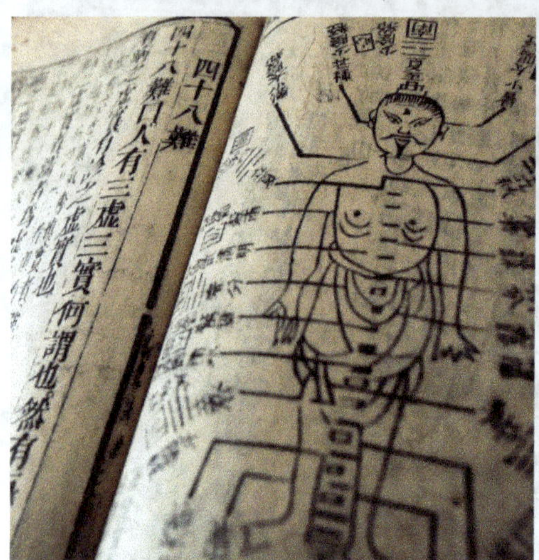
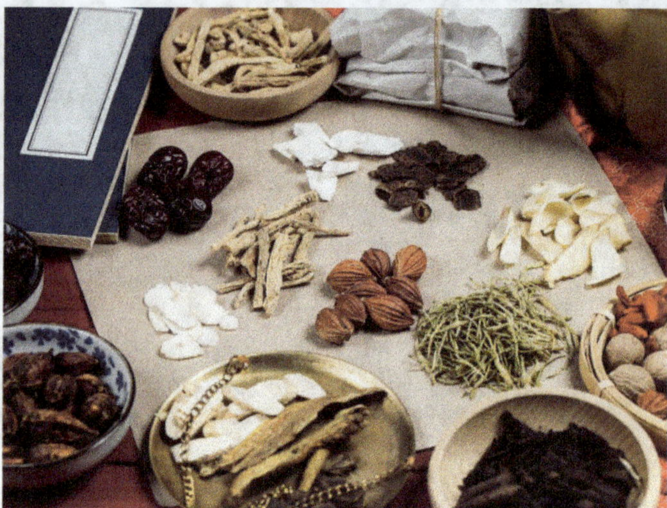

According to TCM, essential oils influence the Shen, which refers to the spiritual essence in the heart that controls consciousness. Ayurveda states that they can enhance the flow of prana, nourish the ojas, and brighten the mental luminosity known as tejas.

TCM and Ayurveda are two of the front runners in holistic medicine systems across the world. They both operate on the principle that we must be in balance, energetically and physically, to create and maintain vitality in our body, mind, and spirit. They both prioritize healthy life force energy and use herbal medicines as the primary source of their medicines.

One of the three treasures in ancient Chinese medicine is known as "Shen" or "The Heart-Mind". Shen is a term commonly used to describe spirit or consciousness. According to this medicine lineage, the Shen resides in the heart, meaning it influences the quality of our thoughts, ideas, senses, emotive responses, and memories.

If the heart is strong and the mind is healthy, this dance gives us the opportunity to experience heightened mental clarity and vitality in our lives. Consider how many expressions we have in just the English language about the figurative heart...

"I have a broken heart"

"I'm wearing my heart on my sleeve"

"I'm having a change of heart"

In Spanish, we have a saying that says "stomach full, heart content", to express the delight after having a delicious meal.

It's said you can see a person's Shen in their eyes and complexion. I'm sure you've had moments when a client walked through your door, and they were either glowing, or you could tell that something was wrong right away; without saying a word.

A person with strong, healthy Shen is a force of love and beauty in this world. Their eyes are bright, their skin is glowing, and their immune system is strong. They are resilient and live in harmony with their environment. They move through obstacles and changes with grace. Their actions reflect clear vision, insight, perseverance and wisdom.

However, when a person is not feeling well and Shen is disturbed, it manifests with dull eyes, dull skin, and you can almost sense the decrease in their life force energy. Their overall vitality appears low.

Aromatics work to harmonize the Shen, or mind of the heart, and assists with Shen disturbances which can range from mild symptoms to severe mental illness such as: anxiety, stress, nervousness, heart palpitations, inability to concentrate, insomnia and psychiatric conditions.

Both physical and emotional stress, traumatic or shocking events, including those that occur in childhood, can disturb the Shen. Through direct inhalation, aromatherapy has a direct bond with the Shen. It stabilizes, nourishes, calms, harmonizes and supports the mind of the heart.

The Body-Mind Connection in TCM:

- The goal is to bring out the expression of emotions, allowing individuals to move forward rather than repressing emotions, which can lead to somatic manifestations in the body.
- Repressed emotions can become pathological and manifest somatically in different parts of the body.
- The intention is to change one's perspective on events, focusing on moving forward rather than dwelling on or reliving negative experiences.
- Choices play a significant role in the healing process, emphasizing the importance of the present moment.
- Blending for mental/emotional states and nourishment in life is essential in TCM.

Aromatherapy Integration:

- Essential oils are used to enhance the process of emotional expression and healing.
- Aromatherapy facilitates easing into change and forming new habits.
- Healing often requires a willingness to change and adapt.
- Essential oils focus on altering one's perception and mindset of the world.
- Vibrational aspects involve changing the frequency of thoughts and the wavelength of how one interacts with the world.
- We can encourage clients to smell each oil and determine which ones they are drawn to, thus providing clues about their emotional profile and desired level of intensity.

Euphoria with Aromatherapy

We all know one of the most delightful feelings there is—is euphoria. This intense feeling of happiness or elation tickles us to our core and gives us a beautiful experience of pure joy.

Aromatics are an incredible tool we can use to invite in this state with our clients. A few oils known for their euphoria inducing properties are: Bergamot, Grapefruit, Lime, Orange, Rose, Jasmine, Nutmeg, Clary Sage, Lavender and Ylang-Ylang.

These oils possess uplifting and calming properties that aid in reducing stress, depression, and anxiety. They also help to uplift the mood, reduce fatigue, and increase energy levels.

Inhaling the aromas from these plants can create a sense of relaxation and contentment almost instantly. And when used with massage and other bodywork treatments— they can ignite a deep state of relaxation. By combining aromatherapy with other relaxation techniques like massage, meditation, and breathing exercises, it is possible to achieve a state of euphoria.

EO's and the Blood Brain Barrier

The blood-brain barrier is a group of compact epithelial cells that stand as our brain's first line of defense against anything foreign or harmful in our blood that does not belong in our brain. In addition to preventing harmful substances from crossing, it also filters out any toxins in the brain back into the bloodstream.

It's primary goal= keep the brain healthy

Now, there are certain nutrients that our CNS (brain and spinal cord) needs—and the BBB has a special set of influx transporters that allow these nutrients to pass through.

When a person suffers from chronic inflammation, neurodegenerative disorders, or oxidative stress— the permeability of the BBB can become compromised. This leads to heightened risk for things like dementia and Alzheimer's later in life. Type 2 diabetes has been recognized as a major player in affecting the BBB's permeability.

That said, the protective nature of the blood-brain barrier can become a major hindrance for transmission of therapeutics to the central nervous system when treating neurological disorders and other conditions.

But what about essential oils?

> "Essential oils of every species cross the blood-brain barrier. This makes them uniquely able to address disease, not only from a physical level, but from a more basic and fundamental level- that of the emotions which are often the root cause of physical illness."
>
> -Dr. David Stewart, Ph.D., R.A

The terpenes, or small lipid-soluble molecules in essential oils, are unique because they can often bypass much of the restrictive nature of the blood-brain barrier. They can swim through the nasal mucosa when inhaled, and also absorb easily into the skin.

This ability makes essential oils very valuable in treating many cognitive stressors and dysfunctions—because they can act directly on the central nervous system easily and effectively.

A meta-analysis investigated the effect of borneol (a terpene-derivative) on decreasing BBB permeability in an experimental model of ischemic stroke in rodents. The study found that treatment with borneol exerted a protective effect by decreasing BBB permeability. The authors propose that borneol improved BBB integrity by:

- Upregulating tight junction proteins
- Accelerating proliferation of endothelial cells
- Acting on cytokines to induce anti-inflammatory effects
- Reducing oxidative reactions
- Improving energy metabolism (Chen et al., 2019)

Anosmia

Total loss of smell is known as "anosmia." And it can be debilitating. We often see people who have suffered from either head trauma or a serious viral infection lose their sense of smell.

Learning to treat anosmia has been a long and arduous process, and many doctors and scientists are continuing to explore ways to support those who have lost this key sense. That said, there has been some really neat research regarding essential oils in treating anosmia.

Check this out:

"For much of history, treating anosmia has been an exercise in futility. Every week for years, Thomas Hummel saw patients at the Smell and Taste Clinic of the Technische Universität Dresden in Germany and sent them home miserable. Some had lost their sense of smell from a head trauma, others following a viral infection. "There's very little that can be done to help them," he says. "That inspired us to find new ways to treat these patients."

Hummel was aware of Wysocki's work and of studies by a German physiologist who had experimented with essential oils decades earlier. So about 10 years ago, he decided to try out an exposure regimen on some patients. He asked 40 anosmic volunteers to sniff four essential oils—rose, eucalyptus, citronella, and clove—twice a day for 12 weeks. Thirty percent of the patients who completed therapy could smell better (The Laryngoscope, 119:496-99, 2009). "That was the first study," says Hummel. "Now, it's been replicated over and over."

The Body

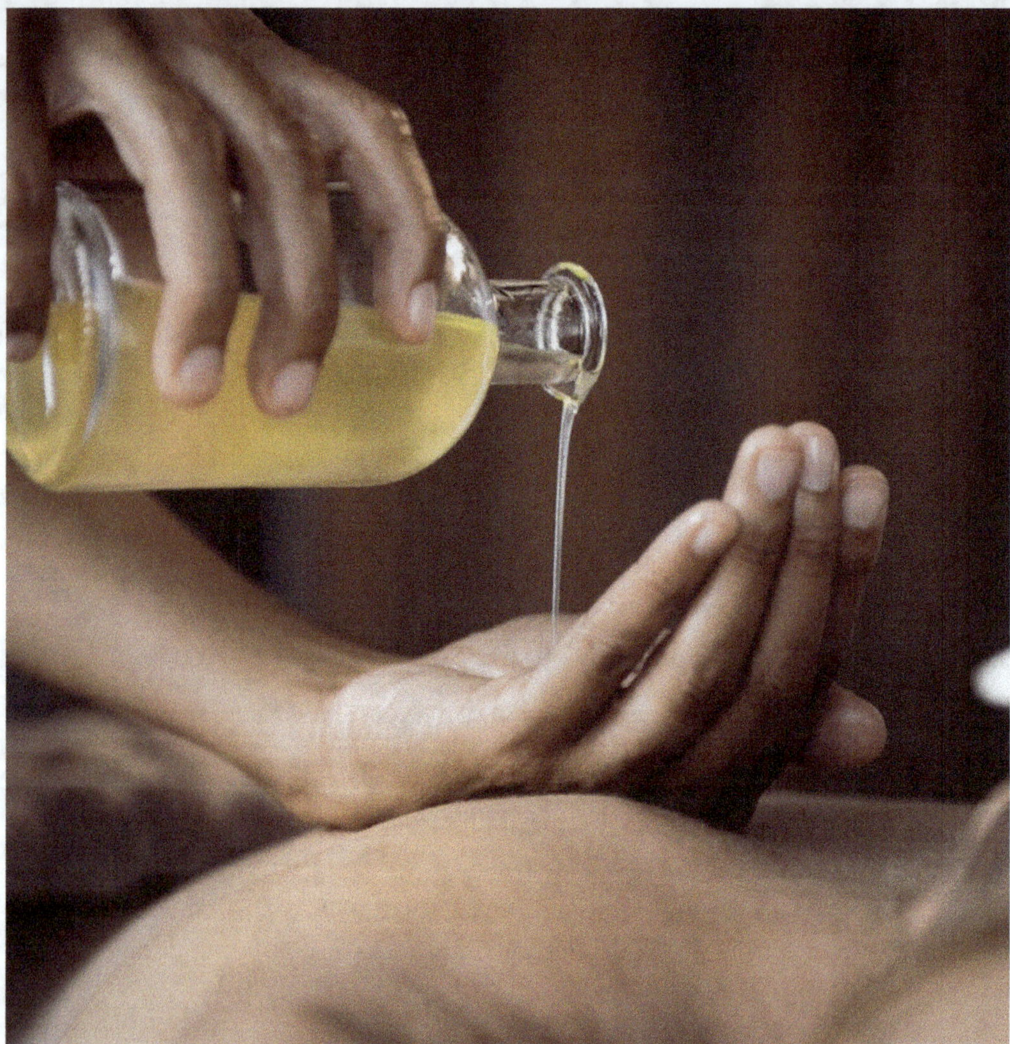

When we apply essential oils topically–they take a journey into our pores, then into the bloodstream as they travel to their designated areas to perform their therapeutic actions.

The oil molecules are so tiny that they swim past the outer layer of the skin (the stratum corneum) then through the dermis, into the capillaries, then into the bloodstream. We can also absorb essential oil molecules through our hair follicles and sweat ducts.

There are many different things that can affect proper absorption, but most notably:

A). The where. Applying oils to the folds of our body (our pulse points) where the skin is more permeable and is closer to our blood and lymphatic vessels is helpful.

B). The state of the skin. Exfoliating dead skin cells and unclogging the pores prior to application increases circulation and helps with proper absorption. Dry brushing and salt/sugar scrubs are great tools for exfoliating.

Essential Oils can help us regain balance by promoting emotional equilibrium and easing physical discomforts. Massage also helps increase the absorption into the skin, which helps to deliver the therapeutic benefit more efficiently.

Internal Use

First things first, do no harm.

The International Federation of Aromatherapists strongly advises against taking Essential Oils internally unless under the supervision of a Clinical Aromatherapist. An exception is when doses of essential oil medications are prescribed by a licensed physician. This is available in certain European clinics, but is rarely available in the United States. People should avoid using essential oils internally, especially if recommended by an untrained individual; and especially if their education is primarily from the marketing perspective rather than clinical.

Plant Affinities

An affinity is a spontaneous or natural liking to something. And plants have a natural liking to, or affinity for, certain systems of our bodies. Traditional herbalists all over the world have the inclination to pinch a leaf, rub it between their fingertips and smell it when they suspect that "there could be a little medicine in there."

Sometimes, just by the aroma, they can predict what the plant might be good for. I've experienced it myself hiking with my dad in the mountains. "This plant must be good for the lungs, ect." And many times after some investigation, we find out that it was pretty accurate that this particular plant has been utilized to support that system of the body.

Disclaimer: This is NOT something I recommend someone to do without proper guidance from an experienced herbalist.

Science has finally been catching up to what traditional herbalists have known all along. They are finding out the "whys" and the "hows". However, families all over the globe do not depend on science to give them permission or confirmation of the power of herbs as medicine. Handed down from generation to generation–the traditions of aromatic plant use have proved themselves time and time again.

Medicinal Action of Herbs

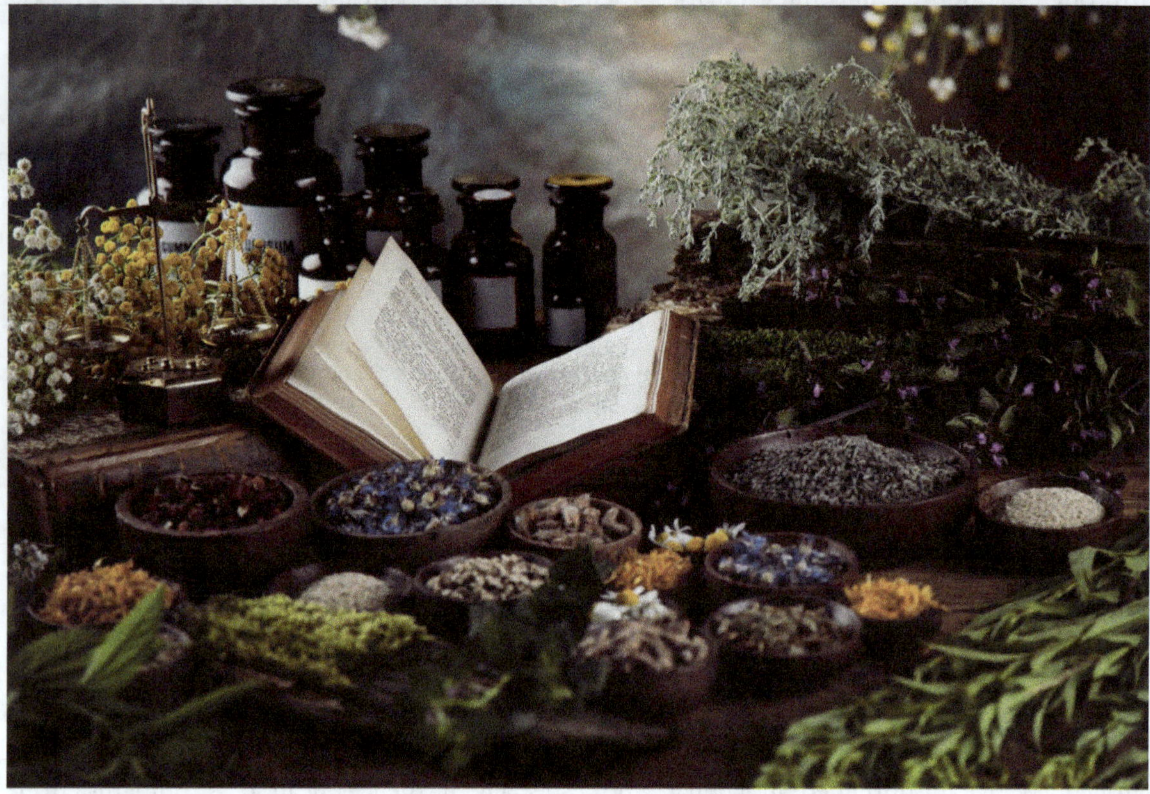

One of the things that is confusing to people, and I'm sure has stumped you a time or two, is the vast range of actions and uses that each herb has to share. Just when you think you have an herb figured out, you learn that it is also used for five new (and sometimes conflicting) things.

How can one plant do all that we read and hear about it? How is it that different herbalists use the same plant for such a variety of different purposes? Why are there so many dissimilarities in the study of herbs?

It's not really as confusing as it may feel. Try this with me. Think about your best friend, or a person you know really well.

Now think about all of the amazing qualities they have. Maybe they're funny, can cook, are a supermom, and can paint or are incredibly creative. And maybe the more you think about it, there are even more layers and qualities that make them an epic person and friend.

Now, if we ask another friend or their partner what qualities they love most about them—they may share an entirely different set of character traits and skills. Maybe it's more of their inner essence and how they are honest, caring, and supportive.

All of this to say—our relationship with plants is as multifaceted as our relationship with people. Each plant is composed of hundreds of different chemicals that make up a complete "personality".

Furthermore, growing conditions influence the personality development plants. And the person, or herbalist, who uses the plant has an influence on the action of the herb. Every relationship is a dynamic dance between two or more beings—and it's no different when you work with plants.

Not to say there isn't a learning curve, or that it doesn't get confusing at times. But it's important to remember plants are not static, inorganic objects—they are living, breathing beings like we are.

So how do we get to know them? By working with them over a long period of time, by listening, reading, studying about them, and, most importantly, using them and integrating them into our lives.

The Spirit (our disposition)

The noun words for "Spirit" in the Greek language are; ru'ahh and pneu'ma. Meaning "breath" but have extended meanings beyond that basic sense. They can also mean wind; the vital force in living creatures; one's spirit, dominant feeling, or disposition.

More than just the impact on the body and mind, essential oils also weave their essence into the unseen parts of us. The way essential oils ground us, affect our emotions, and deepen our sense of calm allows us to sink more into our true nature and remind us we are a part of something so much grander than ourselves.

Here are some ways essential oils impact our spirit:

Emotional Balance: Certain essential oils have been traditionally associated with promoting emotional balance and stability. For example, lavender, chamomile, and bergamot are often used to alleviate stress and anxiety, and promote a sense of calmness, which can positively influence the spirit.

Elevating Mood: Citrus oils, such as lemon, orange, and grapefruit, are renowned for their uplifting and invigorating properties. Inhaling these aromas can stimulate the release of neurotransmitters like serotonin, promoting a more positive and optimistic mood, which contributes to our well-being.

Grounding and Centering: Earthy and woody essential oils, such as cedarwood, sandalwood, and frankincense, are commonly used to instill a sense of grounding and centering. These aromas are believed to connect individuals with their inner selves and foster a deeper sense of awareness.

Emotional Healing: Essential oils are often used in conjunction with mindfulness and therapeutic practices to enhance our inner healing. Resins are what a plant secretes to heal a wound. These oils are often used for healing emotional wounds and traumas. Oils like lavender, frankincense, and patchouli can create a conducive environment for introspection, helping individuals achieve a state of deep concentration and inner peace.

Clarity: Some aromas stimulate the mind and enhance mental clarity. Essential oils like rosemary, clary sage, peppermint and juniper are thought to support mental clarity, allowing individuals to regain mental focus when we need it most.

With this, always consider your client's individual preferences and sensitivities. Personal experiences with scents can vary, so it's advisable to experiment with different oils and observe how each affects your emotional state. Combining aromatherapy with other holistic practices can be especially amplifying.

Aromatherapy Applications

> "The human sense of smell is about ten thousand times more powerful than other senses, and scent travels to the brain so rapidly that the mental or physical response to the fragrance and essential oil emits can be immediate."
>
> — Althea Press
>
> Essential Oils for Beginners: The Guide to Get Started with Essential Oils and Aromatherapy

Aromatherapy Massage

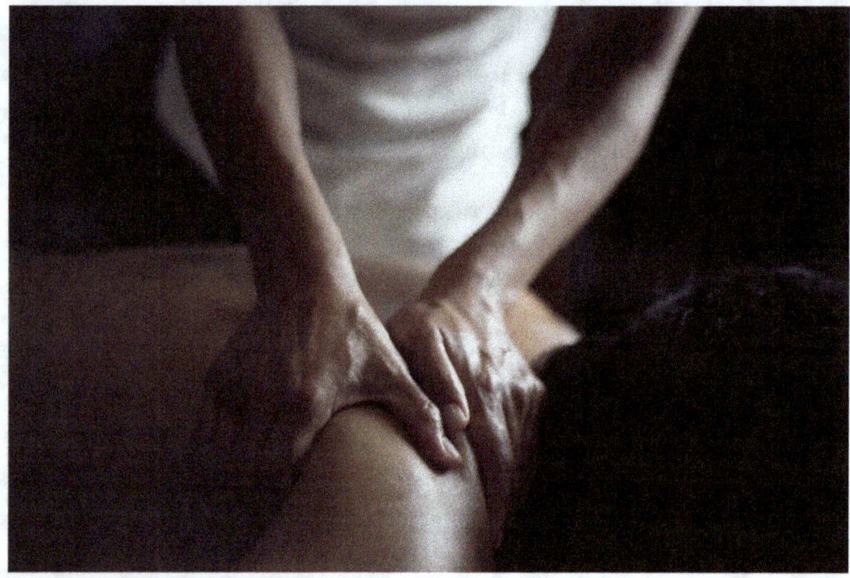

"Aromatherapy without massage is like an orchestra without a conductor,"- Robert Tisserand

Like Tisserand said, aromatherapy and massage go hand in hand, pun intended. And using holistic aromatherapy in your massage practice is something that will elevate your sessions and give your clients more of a holistic healing experience. Not to mention it's fun, practical, and your clients are sure to appreciate this custom curated component of their time with you.

Aromatherapy massage is when we infuse essential oils into our massage oils to help deliver their therapeutic effects. It goes beyond just diffusing the oil in the room, or passing an oil by your client's nose prior to a session.

Aromatherapy massage alleviates pain, helps with chronic fatigue, reduces anxiety and stress, and induces parasympathetic states. It's also one of the most impactful ways to reap the amazing benefits of essential oils.

A true aromatherapy massage links two important senses — smell and touch. This combines the nurturing and therapeutic effects of massage on the soft tissue with the harmonizing effects of the essential oils. Together, they work to bring balance to the body, mind, and spirit.

When we apply an aromatherapy massage blend to the skin, the carrier (or vegetable oil) will remain on the epidermal layer of the skin because the molecules are too large to be absorbed any deeper. The carrier oil functions more as a moisturizer and skin nourisher and protectant.

However, the smaller molecular structure of essential oils allows them to penetrate the dermal layer of the skin and enter the blood vessels. They travel through the circulatory system from here, offering their therapeutic benefit to the muscles and other areas of the body.

Occlusion also allows for greater penetration of essential oils. After applying the essential oils, you can cover the area. This can be with a blanket, wrap, or a warm compress (we will dive deeper into this later).

Pro Tip: Some Aromatherapists give the client a small roll-on bottle of the massage blend they used on them to take home - bringing back the state or feelings they were in when they received their treatments. It's such a charming extra detail and incredibly simple to carry out!

Inhalation

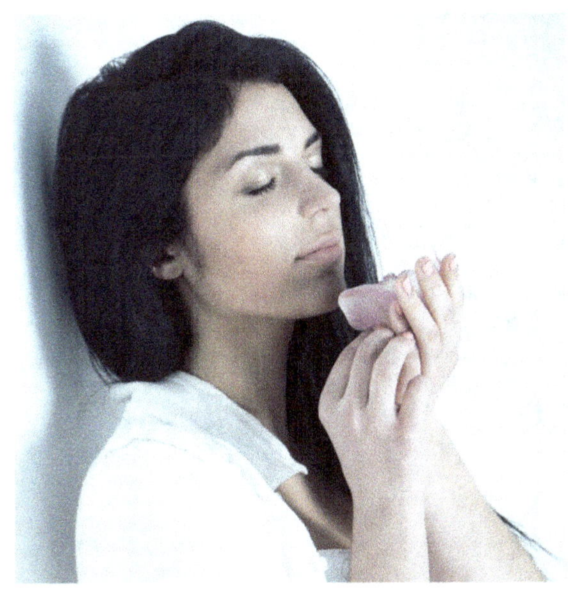

Inhaling the essence of essential oils directly affects the respiratory system and helps with emotional states and neurological conditions because of its direct nose-to-brain route.

This method has a long history of use and is very effective. Consider Vicks VapoRub®, or similar products on the market, made with essential oils and/or constituents (camphor, Menthol, Eucalyptus). The same can be said about topical pain relieving balms, such as Tiger Balm. Despite not being considered an aromatherapy product, people have extensively used these products to relieve pain and respiratory ailments.

Inhalations can also be used to stimulate stored memories.

Inhalation methods

You want to be sure to approach inhalation with caution. These oils are very strong, so the safest way is to apply a drop to a cotton ball or tissue and hold 4-5 inches away from the nose, alternating towards your left and right nostrils, and towards and away from your nose. This will make sure you can experience the different layers of the aroma.

Aromatherapy Inhalers

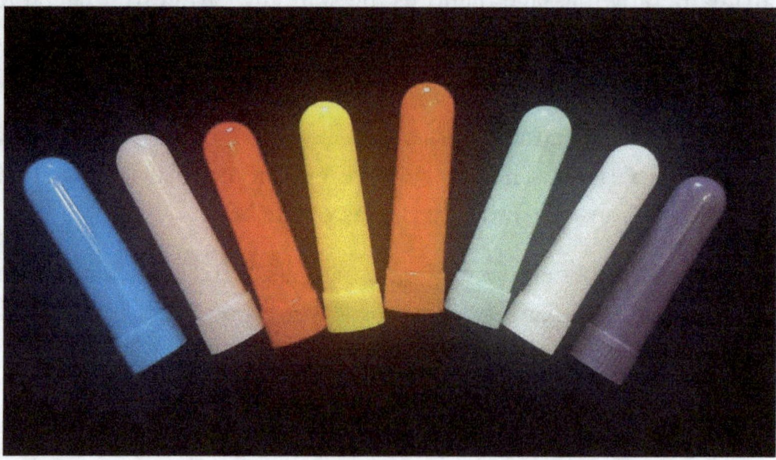

Aromatherapy inhalers are a portable and convenient way to use essential oils when you are on the go. Customizing aromatherapy inhalers for clients takes very little time, making them great gifts!

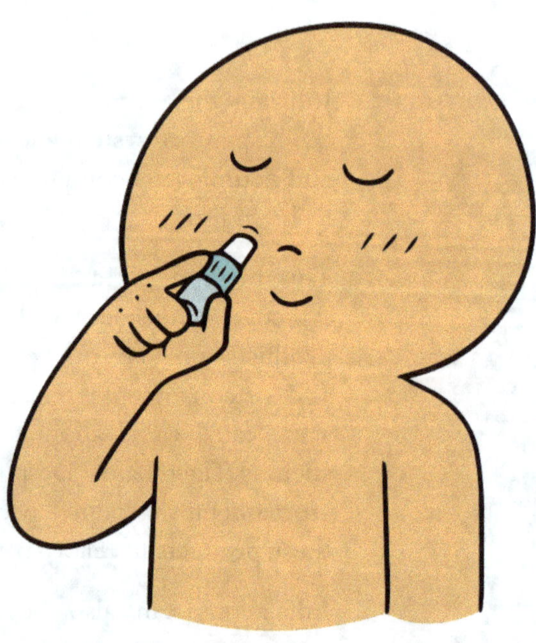

How to Make an Aromatherapy Inhaler

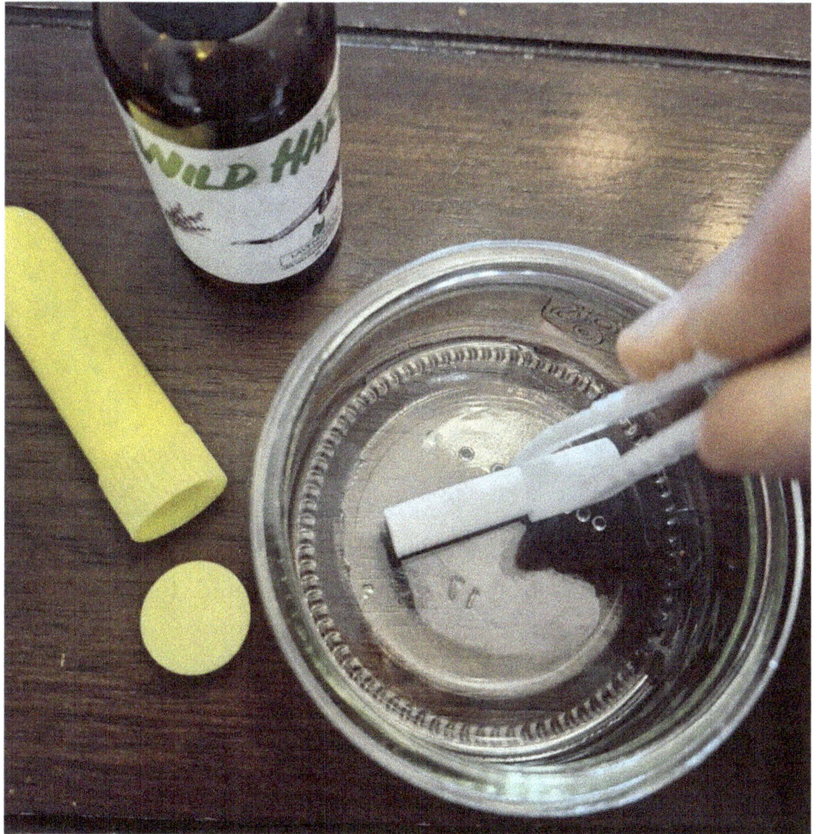

Supplies Needed:

Small dish

Tweezers

Aromatherapy inhaler tube

Directions

Place 15-20 drops of your essential oil combination in the dish

Place the cotton pad in the dish and move it around with the tweezer until it's completely saturated with the oil.

Place to cotton pad into the tube and seal the caps

Your inhaler is ready for use. Can be used as needed or desired throughout the day. Simply remove the cap and hold it approximately 1 inch away from your nose (adjust the distance based on your sense of smell), and inhale deeply.

Steam Inhalation

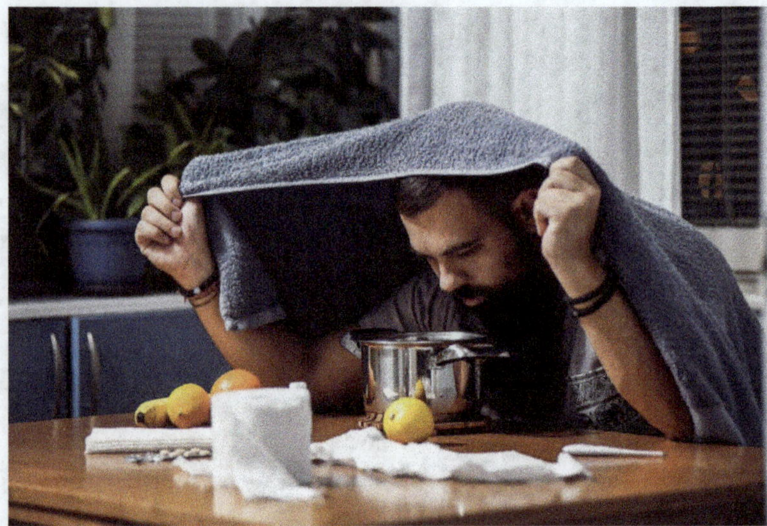

Creating an aromatherapy steam tent for colds using essential oils is a soothing way to ease congestion and promote relaxation. Steam inhalation is specifically tailored for respiratory health and can effectively support the expectorant properties of essential oils. Boyd and Sheppard note that steam inhalation can influence both the volume and composition of fluid in the respiratory tract. They emphasize that using low concentrations of aromatics for brief periods yields the best outcomes. Prolonged exposure can diminish the effectiveness of steam inhalation, hence short durations and low concentrations are key for optimal results.

Steam inhalation is recommended for:

- Relief of upper respiratory congestion (such as during colds or flu)
- Treatment of sinus infections or sinusitis
- Improving respiratory function

Instructions for preparing a steam tent:

Boil 2 cups of water, then reduce heat and let it cool for 5 to 10 minutes.

Pour the water into a glass bowl and place it on a stable surface, allowing the individual to sit or stand comfortably over the bowl.

Add 2 to 5 drops of essential oil or an essential oil blend.

Inhale the steam vapors for 3 to 5 minutes.

Optionally, enhance concentration by covering the head with a towel.

Inhalations can be performed two or three times daily to address specific respiratory issues.

Safety Note: Keep eyes closed during the treatment to prevent irritation. Avoid essential oils that may irritate mucous membranes

Diffusers

Diffusing essential oils is a beautiful way to enliven your space and is one of the simplest ways to receive the plant's benefits on a day-to-day basis. Diffusers have a built-in nebulizer that turns the oil and water into a mist.

Something to note: Experts recommend not diffusing your oils for over 60 minutes at a time. This can cause habituation (olfactory adaptation) and olfactory over saturation. Your body will eventually get used to the aroma, so you cannot smell it anymore, and will not receive any further benefits. Overuse can also cause headaches, nausea, and a feeling of malaise.

Diffuse in 30-60 minute increments, then take an hour break before diffusing again. When around kiddos—diffuse for half of the amount of time.

I love keeping a diffuser in my waiting room, so while my clients are settling in, they are already receiving the relaxing and nourishing benefits of the oils. When diffusing in a public space, it is important to be mindful of others' sensitivities. I prefer to use oils that are most considered "inoffensive" by most, such as those in the citrus family.

Bathing

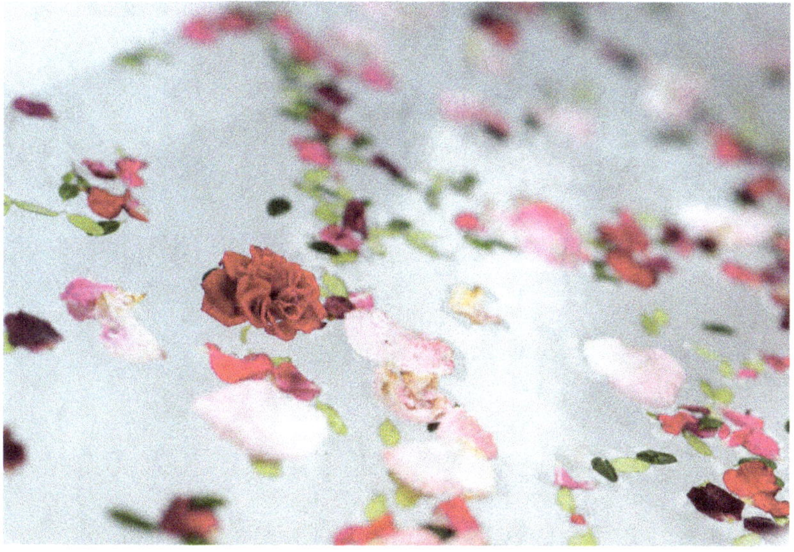

"The way to health is to have an aromatic bath and a scented massage every day."
— Hippocrates

Oh Hippocrates, you idealistic dreamer.

For so many, baths create space for "me" time, allowing us to deeply relax and let the stress of the day melt away. Add some essential oils—and we have got ourselves an incredibly nourishing and healing experience. Next to massage, aromatherapy baths are one of the best ways to receive the numerous benefits essential oils have to offer. Soaking in the essential oil bath blend gives the oils ample time to work by absorbing into your skin, all while you are inhaling the aroma–this will provide physical and emotional effects simultaneously.

Aromatic baths can provide relief from stress and anxiety, help with muscle aches and pains, and can help us get a restorative night's sleep.

To Make a Therapeutic Bath:

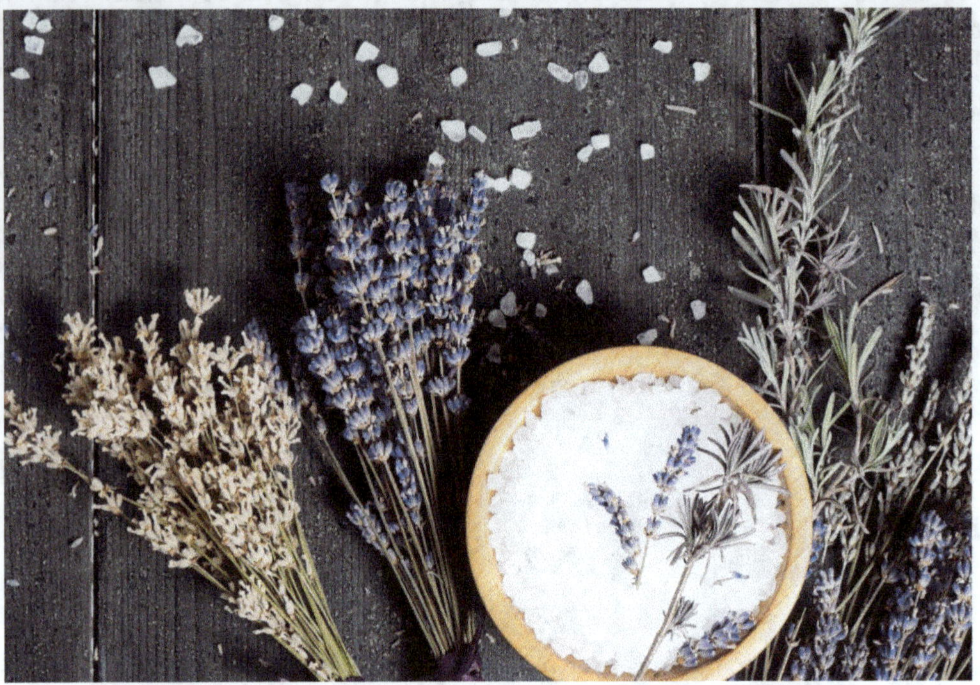

Combine the following in a container. Add to warm bath water. Close the door and soak away the tension for 20 minutes.

- 10-15 drops essential oil (safe for bathing)
- 1 tbsp. Castile soap
- 1-2 cups Epsom salt

A Note on Bath Safety

It is highly recommended to use a dispersant when mixing essential oils and water. You can add a little unscented castile soap or unscented shampoo to your bath blend. Since essential oils are Lipophilic (fat loving) and Hydrophobic (water hating), they are NOT soluble in water. Without a binder, you run the risk of the oil itself coming into direct contact with your skin. Since the oils are so potent, we want to stay away from direct oil-to-skin contact. Direct contact can cause burning and irritation, and can also ignite an allergic reaction for those who do not agree with a particular oil. Read more in the section: Ingredients When Blending Essential Oils and Water.

It is also important to note that not all essential oils are appropriate for use in the bath. Some oils can cause sensitization or are drying and/or irritating to the dermis. To avoid potential skin irritation, it is advised to use fewer than 7-10 drops of citrus oils as a general guideline.

In addition, here are a few more essential oils to leave out of the bath. You may notice many of these oils are derived from plants used in the kitchen, so this is a good way to remember which oils to stay away from when bathing.

- Basil
- Oregano
- Thyme
- Nutmeg
- Cinnamon
- Clove
- Black Pepper
- Lemongrass
- Peppermint
- Bay (Pimenta and Laurus)

Foot Baths

The therapeutic benefits of soaking the feet with herbs, essential oils, hydrosols and salts are powerful. A good foot bath deeply relaxes for the body and mind, and is a perfect way to unwind after a long day.

Maurice Mességué, a French herbalist, acquired fame for his holistic approach to healing with herbs. He believed in the therapeutic properties of plants and was an advocate for herbal foot baths as a method of treating various ailments.

In Chinese medicine, the feet are considered a microcosm of the entire body. According to TCM (Traditional Chinese Medicine), the body has a network of channels (meridians) through which Qi flows. Each channel is associated with specific organs and functions; and the feet hold many acupressure points corresponding to different meridians and organ systems.

Soaking the feet in a warm, essential oil infused bath can bring balance and harmony to the entire system. The warm water relaxes the muscles, opens the channels, and circulates blood and Qi.

Make your foot bath by adding 3- 5 drops of essential oil to a tsp of castile soap. You can also add a handful of Epsom salts to complement. Sit back, relax as you feel the tension melt away.

Bioavailability & Distribution

The bioavailability and distribution of essential oils tells us how much is absorbed and where it goes.

Bioavailability refers to the proportion of a substance that enters circulation and can therefore have an active effect when introduced into the body. Distribution shows us the systems in which a substance affects the body, and at what percentages.

Direct Inhalation (not a diffuser): An average of 50% is absorbed into the blood.

Distribution: Lungs account for 95% and Brain accounts for 5%, followed by the Bloodstream, Liver, and Kidneys.

Topical Use: An average of 5% and up to 10% absorption. Inhalations also occur when applying topically.

Distribution: Skin > Muscle > Bloodstream > Liver > Kidneys

Getting to Know Your Bases

Essential oils are rarely used undiluted. An exception would be to place a drop of lavender on a bug bite to relieve inflammation and itching or tea tree oil on a scratch.

Essential oils are extremely concentrated, so it is recommended to dilute them with a base prior to application on the body. The first step in making any EO product–is to choose your base. Bases include carrier oils, butters, waxes, salts, gels, and more…

Carrier Oils

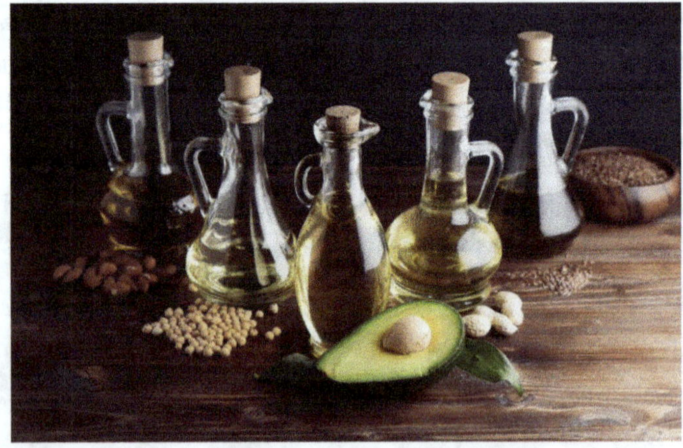

These are fundamental for aromatherapy massage. Carrier oils are vegetable oils extracted from seeds and nuts that are full of nutrients vital for healthy skin. These include essential fatty acids, vitamins, minerals, and antioxidants.

Carrier oils can also be referred to as base oils, and include a variety of different vegetable oils we can use to dilute our essential oils. These oils are high in nutrients like fat-soluble vitamins, antioxidants, and essential fatty acids.

As a general practice, we opt for carrier oils without a scent to ensure the essential oil aroma remains prominent. Certain carrier oils may emit a gentle, nutty scent that is enjoyable to many.

When purchasing carrier oils, seek high quality unrefined vegetable oils. Look for "cold pressed", which means that they are processed at cool temperatures, therefore not destroying vitamins.

Petroleum products such as mineral oils are not suitable for aromatherapy as they are barriers which prevent the skin from breathing and absorbing the benefits of the oils.

Carrier oils can be blended together to adjust the viscosity, or thickness, of a product and to create an optimal base oil for certain skin types. For example–avocado oil is very nourishing. However, it has a heavier viscosity than most other carrier oils. Adding avocado oil to another carrier oil is a common practice to increase the product's ability to nourish the skin.

Let's look at some common carrier oils and their properties:

- Jojoba–A liquid wax with a light, fine texture that is very similar to our body's natural sebum. It absorbs into the skin very well. It has natural anti-inflammatory properties, which are great for soothing eczema, psoriasis, and inflammatory skin conditions. This is a wonderful all-around skin care oil.
- Sweet Almond-a versatile oil that can be used for various purposes and suitable for all ages and skin types. Can be used up to 100% in body or facial oil blends. It is nourishing, non-irritating and is easily absorbed. It has a medium consistency.
- Avocado is rich in skin-nourishing vitamins A and D, potassium and lecithin, omegas, and antioxidants. It is particularly recommended for extremely dry skin. Because of its heavier consistency, it is often used to increase nourishing qualities by blending with other carrier oils.
- Grapeseed– A great all-purpose oil that is suitable for all skin types. It is rich in antioxidants, vitamin C, and fatty acids. It is lightweight and absorbs into the skin easily. The color is light green and the consistency is also light.
- Coconut Oil–Skin protecting Emollient (soothes and softens the skin). Fractionated coconut oil is a fraction of the coconut oil from which almost all the long-chain triglycerides are removed, thus leaving mainly the medium-chain triglycerides and making it an absolutely saturated oil. This saturation gives it a very long shelf life and increases stability. If you need a light oil that mixes well with the other oils, absorbs into the skin easily and will moisturize without clogging pores, then fractionated coconut oil is your go-to oil. It is predominantly composed of Capric and Caprylic acids.

- Apricot Kernel Oil–Skin nourishing and softening, light consistency, great for dry, sensitive, or inflamed skin. Particularly good for facial massage blends because it does not clog the pores and leaves the skin silky and supple. It is rich in oleic and linoleic fatty acids that supply nourishment to the skin.
- Extra Virgin Olive Oil– Nourishing, regenerating, moisturizing, and youth-promoting. A thick and heavier oil that can be used between 10-100% on the body or face. Great for all skin types, particularly dry and mature skin. Contains a natural smell, and can overpower aromas, so keep this in mind when formulating your blends.
- Pumpkin Seed–Deeply moisturizing, high in zinc and vitamin C. Soothing and acts as an anti-inflammatory for the skin.
- Evening Primrose- Deeply moisturizes without clogging pores. Contains the recommended balance of omega 6 to 3 fatty acids. Especially rich in linoleic acid (over 50%), which makes it wonderful for balancing oily, acne-prone skin.
- Camellia Seed Oil (Camellia oleifera)-contains an abundance of natural compounds that your skin will love. This includes Omega 3 and 6 fatty acids, vitamins A, B, C, D, and E. It has a similar molecular weight and composition as our own skin's sebum, absorbing easily into the skin, leaving it silky smooth, and radiant without a greasy feeling. A fantastic oil for a facial massage.
- Hemp Seed Oil- Deeply moisturizes skin without clogging pores. Contains a great balance of omega 6 to 3 fatty acids. Especially rich in linoleic acid (over 50%), which makes it wonderful for balancing oily, acne-prone skin. Hemp seed oil also contains antioxidant vitamins A and E, which help reduce signs of aging and make skin resilient against damage. Hemp seed oil also contains antioxidant vitamins A and E, which help reduce signs of aging and make skin resilient against damage.

Castor Oil

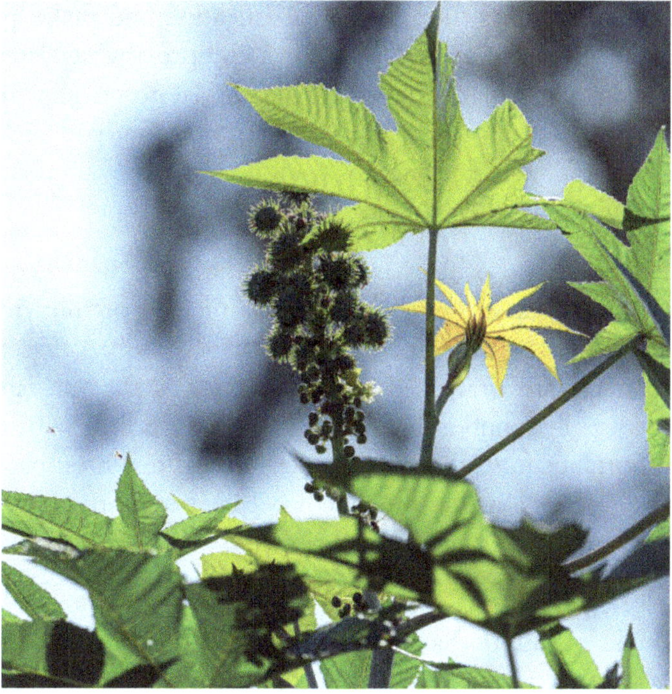

Castor oil has been used for centuries as an effective remedy to treat various ailments. From aiding in digestion to stimulating hair growth, castor oil has multiple uses.

Uncovering the Rich History of Castor Oil

Castor oil is a vegetable oil extracted from the castor bean plant Ricinus communis. Both the plant and its oil have been used for centuries to treat inflammation, infections, and various skin conditions. The Egyptians, ancient Greeks, Romans, and Chinese were all familiar with the natural healing properties of castor oil. In Ayurvedic medicine, it has been used for millennia to cleanse the body of toxins, to boost immunity and improve digestion. It is also known as higuerilla in Latin America.

The active ingredient in castor oil is the ricinoleic acid (up to 90%) found in the beans, which has demonstrated anti-inflammatory properties in laboratory studies. Ricinoleic acid is not found in many other plants or substances, making the castor plant unique since it has a concentrated source. This makes it effective in treating chronic pain, such as joint pains and arthritis. Castor oil supports the body's lymphatic system and may help improve lymphatic drainage, blood flow, thymus gland health and other immune system functions.

Benefits for the Skin

Castor oil is a natural emollient. It supports hydration, repairs, and rejuvenates the skin with its smoothing and softening qualities without clogging the pores. This makes it ideal for reducing the appearance of wrinkles. Castor oil also helps reduce scarring and serves as a treatment for minor cuts, abrasions, and burns, including sunburn.

Exploring the Healing Power of Castor Oil Packs

Using castor oil packs is beneficial for supporting detoxification and make a superb enhancement to your therapeutic massage sessions. A Castor oil pack is a compress which involves applying castor oil to the skin and covering with a soft flannel cloth. Many choose to cover with a sheet of plastic over the area to avoid staining any clothing or furniture. Then a heating pad or hot water bottle may be applied on top of the compress for maximum absorption. The pack is left on for 45- 60 minutes, or overnight, to support detoxification while you sleep.

The liver produces a third to one half of the lymph in the human body. When you compose the lymph produced by the liver and the small intestines, this makes up half of the lymph in the human body. Lacteals are the lymphatic vessels of the small intestine which absorb digested fats. Peyer's patches (aggregated lymphoid nodules) are organized lymphoid follicles that are an important part of gut associated lymphoid tissue usually found in humans in the lowest portion of the small intestine. Peyer's patches establish their importance in the immune surveillance of the intestinal lumen and in facilitating production of the immune response within the mucosa. They act for the gastrointestinal system much as the tonsils act for the respiratory system, trapping foreign particles, surveilling them, and destroying them.

Castor oil packs penetrate deeply, more than just applying it onto the skin alone and will help revitalize the Peyers patches and lacteals, stimulating a "clearing" of the intestinal tract. By supporting these drainage pathways, your body will be better able to detox naturally. Use a castor oil pack to relieve abdominal discomfort, bloating, menstrual cramps, increase circulation and relieve pain from overworked muscles, arthritis.

Unlocking the Amazing Benefits of How Castor Oil Works

- The compression of the pack placed over the liver in combination with the movement of your breathing muscles serves like a pump to your lymphatic system, encouraging lymphatic drainage.
- By placing the pack on your body, its neurological effects on the dermatomes activate the somatic visceral reflexes, triggering the activity of the detoxification organs- liver, kidney, gut, gallbladder.
- The pack stimulates the body's skin receptors, which stimulates the natural oxytocin feedback loop, thus activating the vagus nerve, shifting the body into a rest and digest state where liver detoxification is improved.
- Heat: Using heat allows the castor oil to penetrate up to 6 inches deep into the body.

Conditions that castor oil may help with: Constipation, polycystic ovary syndrome (PCOS), uterine fibroids, endometriosis, cystic breast, benign tumors, muscle and joint aches.

Essential Tips for Using Castor Oil Safely

Using castor oil may have numerous benefits for the skin and hair, but as with any natural remedy, it is important to use it safely. Here are some essential tips for using castor oil:

1. Choose a high-quality product. Use a high-quality oil that is organic, extra-virgin, cold-pressed, hexane-free and in glass.
2. Castor oil should be purchased in a glass bottle due to lipotoxicity.
3. Use appropriate types of cloths for castor oil packs. Castor oil packs should be done with un-dyed fabric like wool or flannel, as cotton can absorb too much of the oil when heated and could potentially cause skin irritation through contact with residue from the oil pack session.
4. Do not apply on open wounds, if the person has a fever or has loose bowels.
5. Avoid if the person has cancer or is undergoing chemotherapy
6. Do not use Castor Oil during pregnancy without speaking to your doctor or midwife first.

How to Use a Castor Oil Pack During Your Massage Session

The best way to apply a castor oil pack is while the client is in a supine position.

1. Apply: the pack first, before massaging the rest of the body. Apply a liberal amount, around 1-2 tablespoons, over the abdomen. Massage the abdomen in a clockwise motion.
2. Cover: with a flannel cloth or 100% cotton fabric: 3-4 layers thick approximately 18X18, enough to cover the treatment area. A cotton flannel pillow case works great for this!
3. Heat: Use a microwavable heat pack, hot water bottle, or any other therapeutic heat source. Check in for comfort. You may use a hand towel between the heat and flannel if desired.
4. Time: Leave the castor oil pack on for a minimum of 20-45 minutes. This gives you plenty of time to work on other areas of the body as the client deeply relaxes with the warm pack.
5. Usually there is little residual oil left, as the body has absorbed most of it. If there is, you can wipe off with a cloth.

Castor Oil Pack Recipes

Essential oils may enhance the effects of your castor oils packs. The following are sample recipes that can be added to 1-2 tbsp of castor oil and applied to the abdomen with your pack.

Blend 1: Belly Blend for Digestion

1-2 tbsp Organic Castor Oil

1 drop Ginger essential oil

2 drops Lavender essential oil

2 drops Lime essential oil

Blend 2: Liver Support Blend - Apply to the right rib cage region.

1-2 tbsp Organic Castor Oil

3 drops rosemary essential oil

3 drops Mandarin essential oil

Blend 3: Nervous System Blend

1-2 tbsp Organic Castor Oil

2 drops Lavender essential oil

2 drops Clary Cage or Chamomile essential oil

Blend 4: Premenstrual Cramps

1-2 tbsp Organic Castor Oil

2 drops Yarrow essential oil

2 drops vetiver essential oil

2 drops Clary Sage essential oil

Salt

Salts can be used as a base to make aromatic products, but your essential oils still need to be blended with a dispersant before adding to your salt bath mixture.

Epsom salt or sea salt baths are excellent for supporting the body by detoxifying physically and emotionally. They enhance the body's immune response by activating healthy blood and lymph circulation, and are incredible for reducing muscular aches and pains.

After a strenuous workout or a long day of walking, a salt bath is the remedy.

Aloe Vera Gel

Aloe vera is brilliant for wound healing, soothing burns, and other tissue damage. Gels make a great medium if you're looking for a non-oily feel with great absorption.

According to Tisserand, aloe vera gel can be an effective carrier in enhancing essential oil absorption. When blended with aloe vera gel, essential oils are more likely to be drawn to the natural oil within our skin and thus be more readily absorbed into the skin than if the essential oil is instead diluted in a lipid-based carrier. When blending, start with a lower dilution of essential oil than you normally would than when working with traditional carrier oils because aloe vera jelly enhances essential oil absorption.

Butters

Butters are another magnificent base for making aromatic products. They are rich, firm in texture–and they feed the skin with nourishing fatty acids, vitamins and antioxidants. Butters are naturally derived from the extracts of seeds, kernels, beans, and nuts.

They also act as wonderful emollients, meaning they smooth and soften the skin. Emollients work by forming a thin hydrophobic film on the surface of the skin that repels water and prevents the loss of moisture. You probably know the incredibly nourishing feeling of applying a luscious body butter after a warm shower. Ahhh…

Butters have an affinity for the skin–meaning they melt on contact with our body temperature while softening and smoothing the skin and hair. They are usually much thicker than creams and lotions because they do not contain water. Another pro of using butters is that they have a long shelf life.

Like many natural products, each butter has a unique profile that acts distinctively by virtue of its unique anti-inflammatory, soothing, moisturizing, or antioxidant properties.

What most butters have in common is that they contain: essential fatty acids, vitamins, proteins, minerals, antioxidants, polyphenols, phytosterols, and tocopherol. They soothe and replenish dry, cracked skin and help to restore aging skin.

That said, butters make an excellent medium to make a cream or massage butter for your treatments!

Cocoa Butter

Cocoa butter is a type of edible fat that is derived from cocoa beans. Cocoa beans are native to South America and are now grown in many tropical regions around the world. The butter is extracted from the beans during the process of making chocolate and cocoa powder.

At room temperature–it is a hard, brittle fat that can be melted to create different aromatherapy products. Cocoa butter is rich in fatty acids, antioxidants and other beneficial compounds that make it a valuable ingredient in skin care products.

Its rich warm scent brings comfort, and it helps the skin retain moisture while nourishing and soothing irritated and/or sensitive skin.

Shea Butter

Shea butter is a fat that is derived from the nuts of the shea tree and is native to West Africa. The butter is extracted from the nuts by a process of roasting, crushing and grinding them into a paste, then compressing the paste to separate the butter from the oil.

Shea butter is rich in skin-loving compounds like vitamins and fatty acids. These compounds protect the skin barrier–and soften and hydrate the skin very well.

We see shea butter used a lot for stretch mark management and as a nourishing scalp and hair treatment. In African traditional medicine–shea butter is used to treat a variety of skin conditions, including eczema, psoriasis, inflammatory skin conditions, and to soothe minor cuts and bites. Adding shea butter to your aromatic formulations leaves you with a silky, powdery feel and is a delightful base for massage and wellness products.

Kokum Butter

Kokum butter is derived from the Garcinia tree that is often used as a thickener for lotions, creams, soaps, cosmetics, and toiletries. Kokum butter by nature is a bit dry and flaky. Because of its hard nature—it does not apply well as a "standalone" application. It is most suitable for being blended with other ingredients to make it more pliable when you are developing body care products.

Kombo Butter (Pycnanthus Angolensis)

Kombo butter is harvested and cold pressed from the seeds of the tropical West African tree. This beautifully dark and rich butter absorbs easily into the skin and works wonders on dry or irritated skin.

It's also high in myristoleic acid, which is why we believe it is used traditionally for pain relief. It can be combined with other butters and carrier oils to make your muscle and joint care blends!

PRO TIP: This butter may stain light clothing— so be sure to dab off any excess butter from your skin so it doesn't get on your clothes.

Refined vs Unrefined Butters—What's the Difference?

Refined butters have gone through a process to remove the odor, which results in a creamy white or off-white color and milder scent. The refinement process gives butters a longer shelf life, but you lose a lot of the nutrient dense magic.

Unrefined aka raw/crude butter retains its natural color, aroma, and all of its original properties because it has not been processed. Unrefined butters are considered more pure and may contain more nutrients (including vitamin E and fatty acids) and healing properties than refined butters.

Waxes

Beeswax (Cera flava)

We love our bees!

Beeswax is a natural wax made from the honeycomb produced by bees and is a go to ingredient in beauty products. You've probably used it in a lip balm before.

Beeswax has a wide range of benefits, and it's a great way to add firmness to butters and salves to create a more balm-like texture.

It is also a humectant—meaning it helps retain moisture on the skin. It's incredibly nourishing for dry and chapped skin, and is a natural anti-inflammatory and anti-bacterial.

Use this wax to add firmness to your balms, salves, butters, and other body care blends. As you melt beeswax, the warm scent of honey becomes stronger and fills the room! Blend a richly textured topical salve or butter with beeswax, which will linger on your skin longer than a more absorbent lotion or oil.

Beeswax has a melting range of 144 to 147 °F (62 to 64 °C), therefore if you replace it with a wax of a higher melting point, you usually need less. Beeswax is also an emulsifier so it makes ointments less 'oily' and more easy to absorb.

Overall, beeswax is a versatile ingredient used in many products for topical use– and provides natural moisturizing, healing and protective properties for the skin. You might be able to purchase beeswax from your local bee keeper.

Carnauba Wax

Carnauba wax is a great natural (and vegan!) wax that is commonly used in cosmetic and personal care products–including salves. The "Tree of Life" or Copernica cerifera is the species of palm from which people harvest Carnauba wax. These indigenous trees flourish in northeastern Brazil and are a different species than the palms planted purely for their oil.

Harvesters derive the wax from the leaf of the tree and perform manual pruning once a year, which allows the tree to continue growing for decades.

We often see Carnauba wax used:

1. As a natural thickening agent: Carnauba wax is often used in salves to thicken the mixture, giving it a more luxurious, spreadable texture.
2. To improve consistency: The unique properties of carnauba wax give it the ability to help improve the consistency of a salve, making it easier to apply and spread.
3. For its emollient properties: Carnauba wax has emollient properties that can help soothe and soften skin. This makes it an excellent ingredient for salves that are designed to treat dry or irritated skin.
4. To protect against moisture loss: Carnauba wax creates a protective barrier on the skin, helping to prevent moisture loss. This can help to keep the skin hydrated and prevent dryness and flakiness.

The melting range of carnauba is 82–86 °C (180–187 °F). When using Carnauba wax, use ¾ to ½ the amount of beeswax called for in most recipes.

Ex: If a recipe says 10g beeswax, replace it with 5-7.5g Carnauba wax.

Candelilla wax (Euphorbia antisyphilitica)

Candelilla wax is another vegan vegetable wax obtained from the leaves of the Candelilla shrub (Euphorbia cerifera), native to northern Mexico and the southwestern United States. It is a yellowish-brown, odorless wax with a unique composition that makes it a popular ingredient in cosmetic and personal care products.

Candelilla wax is a lovely plant-based alternative to beeswax–making it a great option for those following a vegan lifestyle.

Candelilla wax acts as a barrier when applied to the skin, locking in moisture and preventing dryness. This can help promote healing in dry or chapped skin, which is why we see it used mostly in salves. It is also an emollient, which means it helps to soften and smooth the skin.

It's firm and has a high melting point, which helps to solidify and stabilize the formulation of salves, preventing it from melting too easily and ensuring it remains solid at room temperature.

Candelilla wax also contains compounds that possess natural antibacterial and antimicrobial properties, which help protect the skin from harmful bacteria and reduces the risk of infection with minor cuts, wounds, and abrasions.

The melting range for candelilla wax is higher than beeswax 155.3–162.5 °F(68.5–72.5 °C).

When formulating with candelilla wax, use half the amount of beeswax in the recipes.

Ex: If a recipe says 10g beeswax– replace it with 5g candelilla wax.

Ingredients When Blending Essential Oils and Water

As we all know–oil and water do not mix. Essential oils are oil-soluble and "hydrophobic" which means that they can't be incorporated into an aqueous medium.

A dispersant is needed to create a blend that contains essential oils and water.

Grain Alcohol (ethanol)

Alcohols are able to kill many types of bacteria on the molecular level. Tisserand states: "Ethanol (ethyl alcohol) is a 'cidal' agent capable of killing microorganisms. It can be used to eliminate microbial contamination and prevent microbial growth. It is also a solvent capable of dissolving oils. As such, it's suitable to use as a solubilizer when dissolving small amounts of volatile essential oils."

When making a spray, the percentage of ethanol that's part of the total of the spray formula needs to be a minimum of 20-30%.

What alcohol to use? You don't want to use just any cheap vodka- which usually is 80 or 100 proof or only 40-50% ethanol content and therefore will not properly solubilize essential oils.

In the event that 190 proof (95%) grain alcohol is not available, one can use Everclear 151 proof (~75%), but it may not solubilize essential oils as easily.

Solubol

Solubol is a natural, alcohol-free dispersant that effectively disperses essential oils in water. Its mild aroma doesn't influence the scent of your oils. It is recommended to use a ratio of 1 part essential oil to 4 parts solubol. Blend, then add water or hydrosol to fill the bottle, cap the bottle and shake gently to disperse the essential oils into the water or hydrosol.

Castile Soap

Made from natural vegetable oils–castile soap is a great ingredient for making soaps, cleaning products, shower gels and other "cleansing" aromatherapy products. Castile soap is gentle, cleanses the skin without stripping away its natural oils or causing irritation, and is a great option for people with allergies or sensitive skin.

A big plus–castile soap is eco-friendly and is made from natural ingredients. It's bioavailable and doesn't contain any synthetic chemicals that can harm the environment. Overall, it's a beautifully natural and versatile ingredient for aromatherapy products. When making a bath blend, you can add 1 tablespoon of castile soap to help disperse essential oils in the bath water.

Infused Oils

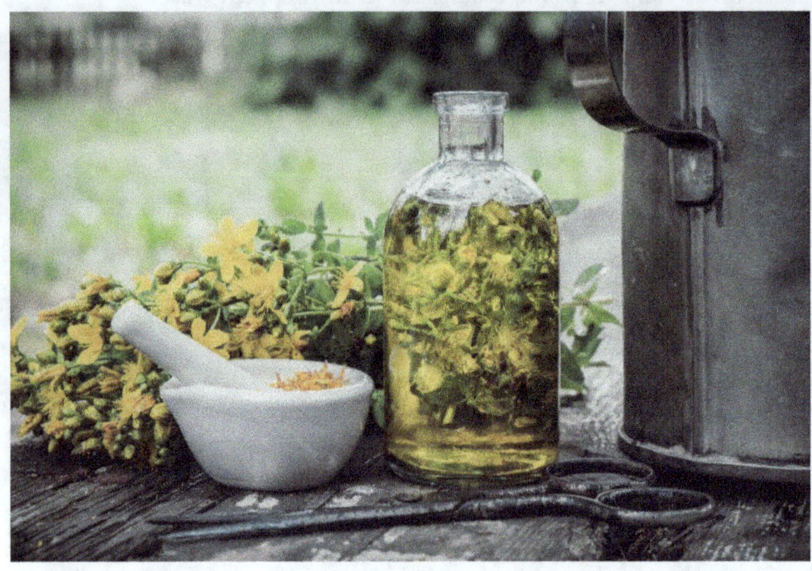

Infused oils are carrier oils infused with the essence of your choice of herbs. They make fabulously versatile ingredients you can use to make many products like soaps, butters, body oils, lip balms, gels, and salves. You get a double dose of goodness with infused oils because they carry the healing properties of both the herbs used, and the vegetable carrier.

They are also incredibly easy (and fun!) to make.

Fixed oils such as fractionated (MCT) coconut oil, almond oil, and olive oil are the most popular oils used for infusion. These work as the solvent in the recipe, which is the extracting material used to draw out the beneficial properties of the plant. They have the longest shelf lives and are suitable for many different applications. That said, you can use any vegetable carrier oil you like.

When infusing, I always recommend using dry plant material. Using fresh plant material puts you at risk of losing your batch to mold or bacteria growth.

One exception is St. John's Wort (Hypericum perforatum)—which needs to be infused using his freshest buds on a warm sunny day.

If your final product does not have a strong, robust aroma that slaps you after opening the jar, that is normal! Most herb oils have a light, subtle aroma. They will not necessarily have a strong aroma or contain the same properties as the essential oil. This is because fixed oils, though a useful solvent for extracting the plant's properties, do not sufficiently extract the volatiles.

Remember, essential oils are extracted through steam distillation and expression. However, to enhance the fragrance and the properties of your herb infused oil (depending on the intention of your blend), you can add the appropriate amount of essential oil(s) to the finished product.

Infusing your own oils is a great way to get creative with herbal blends. Try intuitively combining different herbs with your carrier oil of choice, and see what happens. I love infusing lavender, rose and chamomile flowers in jojoba oil to make a super relaxing massage oil.

What herb/oil combo are you thinking of trying out first?

Pro tip: After straining, fine herb sediment can make your oil a bit gritty—if this bothers you, strain again through a coffee filter.

Common Herbs Used for Infusing

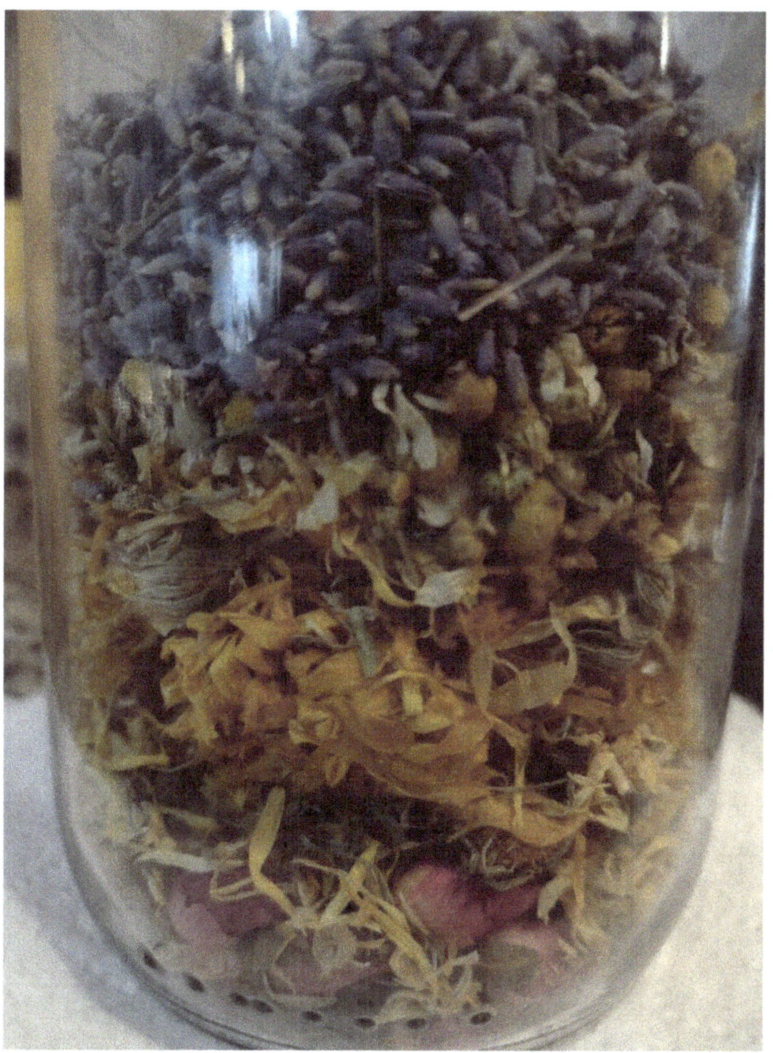

Calendula (Calendula officinalis)

Calendula is a miracle herb for the skin. It's cooling, acts as an antimicrobial, anti-inflammatory, and antifungal; and is a superb vulnerary herb—a plant used to treat wounds.

Clinical studies have shown that calendula increases cell proliferation, is bacteriostatic, and encourages the body to heal at a proper pace. It has a specific affinity for swollen, hot, painful, pus-filled tissue—so it's perfect for nastier wounds.

Use calendula infused oil for wounds, dry skin, ulcers, cracked skin, rashes and any other skin ailments. Calendula is very popular as a main herb in healing salves for breastfeeding mamas and babies as well.

Arnica *(Arnica montana)*

Arnica is a powerful herb for joint pain, muscle pain, inflammation, and bruising. When you think of Arnica—think pain relief.

The first documented medicinal use of the fresh or dried flowers of arnica dates back to the 1500s. The flowers were used to create poultices for treating sprains and bruises, aches and pains, and to stimulate blood flow.

Arnica is also a popular holistic treatment for body pain caused by trauma or surgery. It helps decrease swelling from sprains, muscle strains, and broken bones.

Arnica infused oil makes a great massage oil for your older patients who suffer from joint pain, osteoarthritis, and stiffness.

St. John's Wort *(Hypericum perforatum)*

St. John's wort is a timeless herb that is most well-known for treating depression and uplifting the mood by increasing the levels of certain neurotransmitters—such as serotonin, dopamine, and norepinephrine in the brain.

Physically, its antibacterial and anti-inflammatory properties make it a popular ingredient in mainly ointments and creams developed for wound healing and skin irritation. Great for regional nerve pain when applied topically. Helpful for sciatica, lower back pain and carpal tunnel syndrome. The oil can be used to treat bruises, varicose veins, and mild burns, including sunburns. Dioscorides, the most famous herbalist of the ancient Greeks, mentions the use of St. John's Wort for sciatica and other nerve problems. So do many other ancient Greek healers. Theophrastus recommended it for external wounds and cuts; Pliny recommended taking it in wine for poisonous reptiles; and it was included in the materia medica of Galen and Paracelsus.

Remember, St John's Wort is the exception for infusing—you want to infuse the fresh buds rather than the dried flowers.

Caution: may cause photosensitivity in some individuals. If you get a rash, itchy or red skin, discontinue using it.

Chamomile *(Matricaria recutita)*

Chamomile= soothing. You've probably had chamomile tea to wind down from a long day or to help you sleep. It helps soothe the spirit, relax the body and mind, and supports digestive health by relaxing the muscles in the stomach.

It's best friend–lavender. You can make an incredibly relaxing base for your massage oils and butters by combining chamomile and lavender with almond oil (or your favorite carrier). This base is suitable for your clients who are particularly stressed.

There are two common types: Roman and German chamomile. German chamomile contains an abundance of Azulene, a constituent responsible for its beautiful blue color that will be released during distillation. They have similar properties–though German chamomiles compounds make them especially great for wounds and skin conditions.

Babies love it too! Chamomile based creams are fantastic for treating diaper rash.

Comfrey *(Symphytum officinale)*

Also known as "knit bone," people have been using this herb for centuries to treat a variety of pain and inflammation related issues and to speed up the healing of fractures.

Think of Comfrey like combining the power of Calendula and Arnica.

Comfrey roots and leaves contain allantoin, a substance that helps new skin cells grow, along with other substances that reduce inflammation and keep skin healthy. Among its clinical uses, comfrey can help relieve pain, reduce inflammation of muscles and joints, speed the healing of bruises and contusions and potentially aid in the treatment of fibromyalgia.

In the U.K., researchers found that practitioners prescribed it in about 15 percent of all consultations regarding tendon, ligament and muscle problems, fractures and wounds. Use on unbroken skin.

Cayenne *(Capsicum annuum)*

Yes, the pepper! Cayenne peppers have an ingredient called capsaicin, a compound that gives them "heat".

Applied topically–capsaicin can help to ease pain by reducing the amount of a neuropeptide known as substance P that travels to the brain to signal pain. With less substance P, feelings of pain decrease.

Vanilla bean *(Vanilla planifolia)*

A luxurious and comforting treat that will add warmth to the heart. The aroma has an intensely soothing effect. I like to use jojoba or almond oil when infusing my personal batch of this special creation, but you can also get creative by using other carrier oils of your choice.

Kava Kava (Piper methysticum)

Pacific Islanders have praised kava Kava for centuries, using it internally to calm nerves and help with relaxation. This anxiolytic herb promotes natural relaxation and helps in coping with stress. It can be highly sedative and has been known to numb certain body parts of the body. Traditional herbalists have used Kava as a reliever of pain, inflammation, tension and spasms.

Topical benefits: The infused oil of Kava used topically deeply relaxes the muscles and takes the "fight" out of them. Add rose petals to create a beautiful heart- calm synergy.

How to Make an Infused Oil

"The Folk Method" With Dried Herb

Fill a clean and sterilized jar with dried calendula flowers, or other dried herbs, until the jar is full. Gently press flowers down to fill the jar as much as possible– but don't press too hard.

You want the oil to be able to move around and between the plant material. Cover dried flowers with your carrier oil of choice. Organic extra virgin olive (Olea europaea), sunflower oil (Helianthus annuus, sesame oil (Sesamum indicum), jojoba oil (Simmondsia chinensis), and sweet almond oil (Prunus amygdalus) are some of my favorites.

Solar Method (slow)

If you're not in a hurry, the solar method, or windowsill method, is super easy. Pour your herbs and oil into a glass jar. Make sure you put enough oil to cover the herbs. Label and set in a sunny window. Shake your jar daily. Let the mixture infuse for a minimum of 2 weeks (4-8 weeks is best).

Then press out oil with an herbal press or use a cheesecloth. Compost the herbs and store your infused oil in a glass jar with a label and date.

Stove Top Method (Fast)

For this method, pour the mixture (flowers and oil) directly into a double boiler pot. Use enough oil to cover the herbs completely about 2-3 inches over the top of the herbs. Gently heat the water in the bottom pot until it is simmering. Make sure the oil does not get above 110 degrees F. Allow the oil to infuse for 4 to 8 hours.

Remove from heat and let the oil cool down to room temperature. Press the oil, store in a clean glass jar, and label. Herbal oils, depending on the carrier you use, can last 2-4 years when stored properly.

The Slow Cooker Method (not fast, not slow)

This method is quicker than the sun method, but not as quick as the stovetop method. You can set this one up and let it do its thing while you sleep!

What you'll need:

A slow cooker with an adjustable temperature dial or a 'keep warm' setting that stays around a temperature of about (145 to 165 F) 62 to 74 C.

- 4 parts oil
- 1 part dried herb

Place your herb and oil in a heatproof mason jar with the lid on, and place in a slow cooker with a couple of inches of water. Do not put on the slow cooker lid. Put on 'keep warm' and leave on overnight.

In the morning, strain the herbs, reserving the oil. You can then repeat the infusion with a new batch of herbs if you want or bottle the oil. Don't forget to label and date.

Infused Oil Recipes

Pain Relief Infused Oil

- 1 part Arnica montana
- 1 part Comfrey (root and/or aerial parts)
- 1 part Calendula
- 1 part St. John's Wort
- 4 parts carrier oil of choice
- 5 ml (1 tsp.) castor oil for each 25 ml of the above blend

Essential Oil Synergy - for Pain Relief Infused Oil

For each ounce (2 tbsp./30 ml) of the above carrier, add the following essential oils:

- Eucalyptus: 2 drops
- Frankincense: 3 drops
- Copiaba: 2 drops
- Roman Chamomile: 3 drops
- Ginger: 3 drops
- Rosemary: 3 drops
- Lavender: 3 drops

Flower Power Infused Oil

This recipe will produce a luxurious infusion with a mild aroma of gentle flowers that have an affinity for the skin and powerful skin healing properties. Use this infusion to make formulations that will soothe and nourish the skin like butters, salves and body oils.

Infused with Jojoba, Almond, Apricot or your preferred carrier(s).

- 1 Part Lavender buds
- 1 Part Chamomile flowers
- 1 Part Rose Petals
- 1 Part Calendula Flowers

Vanilla Bean Infused Oil

Vanilla infused jojoba oil is divine. This will produce a luxurious infusion that will add an extra bit of magic to your body butters.

Recipe:

- o   16 oz jojoba oil or sweet almond oil or apricot oil (or all 3!)
- o   5-6 organic vanilla beans
- o   Double boiler
- o   Love and patience

How to:

Cut your vanilla beans vertically and throw the seeds into your jojoba oil. Then cut the vanilla beans into smaller pieces and place them into the oil.

Using a double boiler, put about 1 cup of water in the bottom pot and your vanilla/jojoba mixture into the pot on top. Set the stove's temperature at low and allow it to simmer.

Remember: It's about simmering and not wanting to boil the oil. Simmer for around 3 hours per day until you are happy with the aroma. After 2-3 days, the oil will become infused and you can strain it through a cheesecloth.

There might be tiny vanilla seeds in the oil after straining. Don't let them go to waste! Pour carefully without pouring all of it into one jar, leaving some behind so you can use this as a gentle facial exfoliant or blend with body scrub recipes later on.

Cayenne Infused Oil

Follow the instructions on making an infused oil using one of the methods above. It will be difficult to strain out the cayenne powder so you can let it settle at the bottom and try to leave it there or you can strain it through a muslin cloth. Use this oil to make a salve to relieve sore muscles and joints. Great for localized pain relief.

- 4 oz olive oil or other carrier oil
- 1 tbsp Cayenne powder or flakes

Kava Kalm

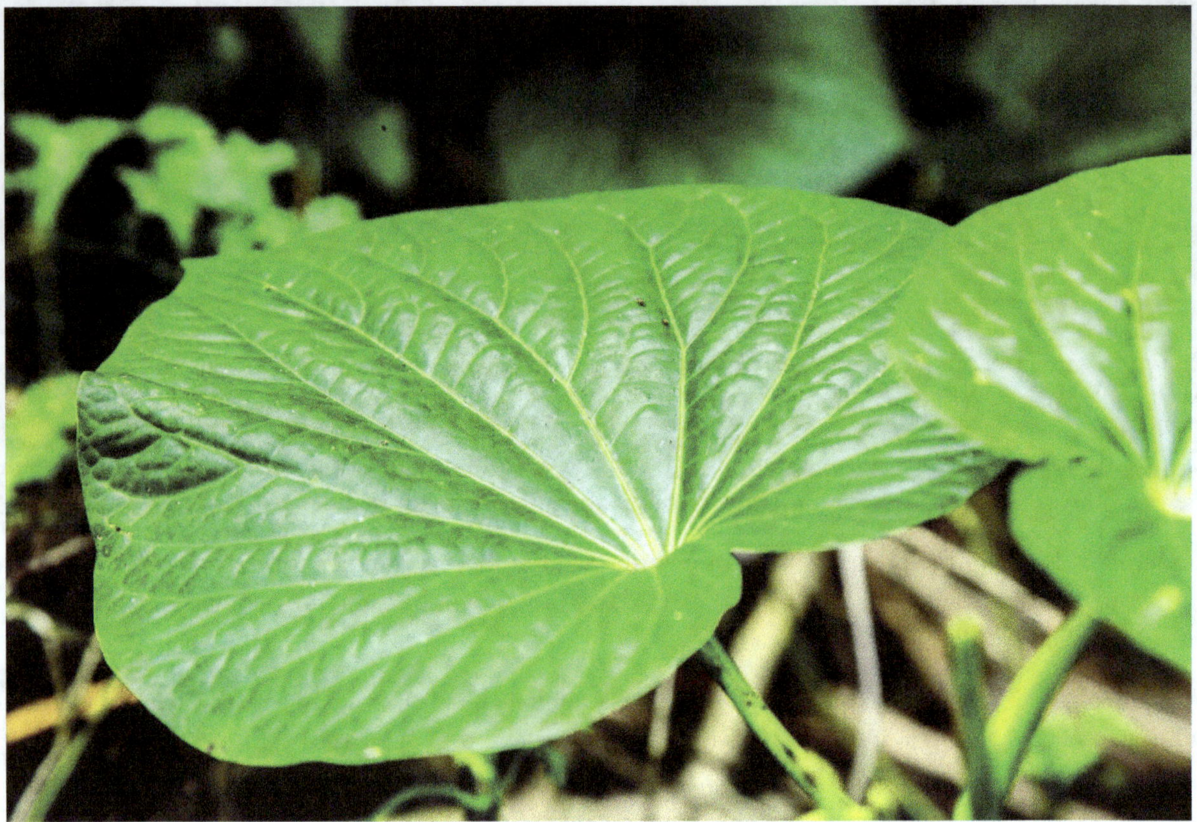

This exquisite oil tranquilizes an agitated nervous system, or as I like to say, when your nervous system has taken a beating. This often manifests as tense, spastic muscles with the inability or difficulty to relax and "let go".

- 15 ml Kava Infused oil
- 15 ml Fractionated coconut oil (or other carrier oil of choice)
- 4 drops Clary sage
- 2 drops Ylang ylang
- 4 drops Bergamot

Butters, Balms, and Salves

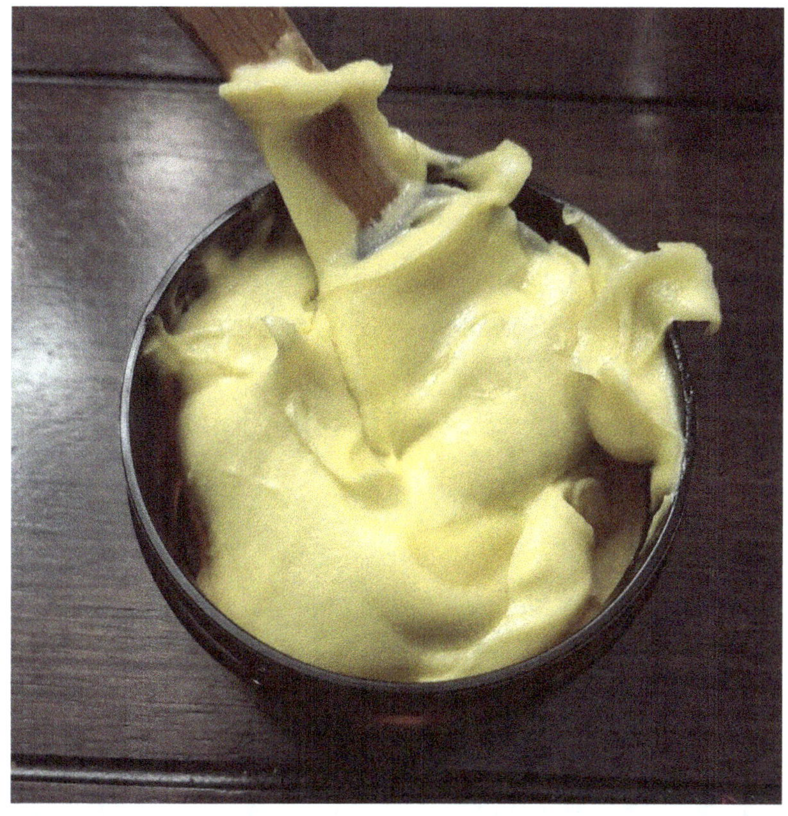

There are so many creative ways we can incorporate essential oils and the power of aromatherapy into our bodywork practices. It's incredible when you feel empowered to make your own products and to make products with your clients in mind.

Butters, balms, and salves are three incredible allies for us as bodyworkers. Our ability to combine botanical extracts, essential oils, and nourishing carrier ingredients allows us to craft indulgent and supportive products for our clients.

These rich and thicker products are phenomenal particularly for the skin–to nourish dry or cracked skin, to treat specific skin conditions and wounds, and to protect the skin from environmental irritants. They are great for localized treatment where pain, inflammation, and stiffness are present.

You can create these products to send your clients home with as samples to use in between sessions, and you can also custom make them a product to purchase.

What's the Difference?

A butter is a combination of essential oils or infused oils with a carrier butter like shea, cocoa, or kombo butter. Really nourishing for dry skin, and super soft and creamy in texture. They are more light and spreadable in consistency than a balm or salve.

A salve is a semi-solid ointment that combines waxes with carrier oils, infused oils, and/or essential oils. Wonderful for healing wounds, soothing damaged skin, and can be used to treat specific conditions. Salves tend to be more thin and oily in consistency than a balm, making them easier to spread.

A balm is firmer than a salve and they act more as a protective barrier against environmental irritants. Balms typically have a longer shelf life than salves and also have a waxy base.

A General Guide

You can easily adjust the consistency of salves depending on your preferences. Use less beeswax for a softer salve and more beeswax if you'd like a firmer salve.

Making Butters, Balms, and Salves

The Stovetop Method

Use this as a general guide when creating your balms and salves.

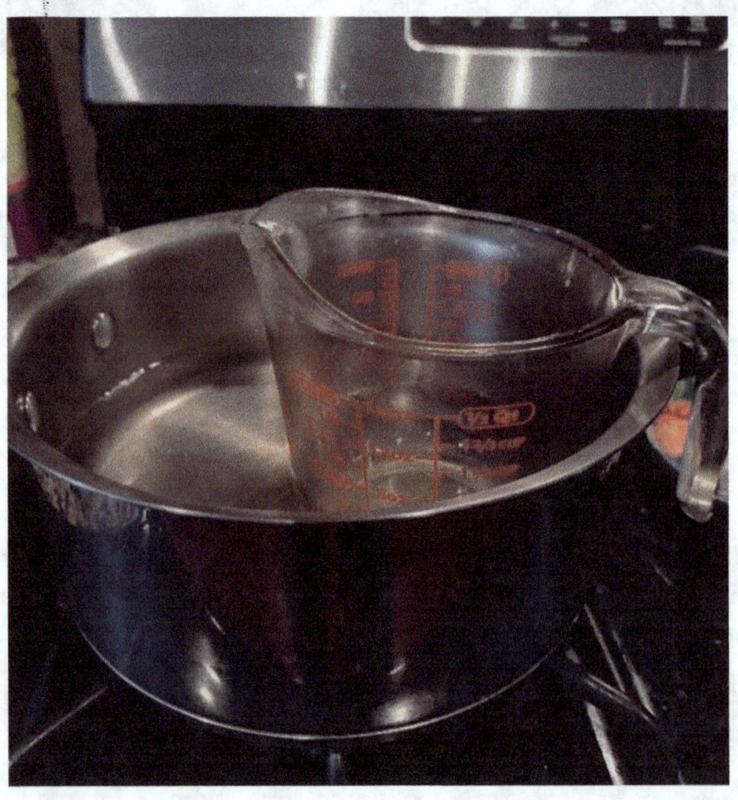

- Have all of your ingredients weighed and ready.
- Fill your pot 1/4 of the way with water and bring to a low submarine boil.
- Place a pyrex measuring cup in the pot of water so the water heats the outside, and the handle is hanging over the edge of the pot. You can also use a double boiler.
- As the water heats up, make sure it doesn't boil too strongly, so that water falls into the Pyrex. We need to keep water out of your product!
- First, place the beeswax (if your recipe calls for beeswax) in and allow it to melt almost completely. Stir occasionally with the back of a metal spoon or stirring rod.
- Mix in your herbal oils or carrier oils and stir occasionally until the beeswax is melted.
- Remove from heat.
- Add essential oils and pour in your sterilized container.
- Pour the blend in glass jars or tins and cover.

Butter Recipes

Whipped Massage Butter (heatless)

This recipe does not require a heat source and you can make it in a short amount of time. It creates a luxurious, soft butter ideal for massage or as a moisturizer.

- 4 oz shea butter
- 1 tbsp (13g) carrier oil of choice
- 40 drops essential oils (optional)

All you need is an electric mixer–simply blend your ingredients in a bowl. Begin with 1 tbsp of whichever carrier oil you're using. If you prefer a lighter consistency, gradually add oil until you reach your desired consistency.

Foot & Reflexology Butter

- 3 oz shea butter
- ¼-½ oz castor oil

Using the stove top method::

- Add castor oil and shea butter into the Pyrex to melt. Stir occasionally with the back of a mental hospital or stirring rod.
- Be sure to stay by the stove until melted. You do not want to overheat the shea butter.
- Once melted–remove with a mitten, pour into a glass jar, and cover.

If you decide to add essential oils, do this last, right before pouring in a jar or directly in the individual jars.

- Store in the fridge initially to speed up solidification

Skin Silk Butter

A firm, multi-purpose butter. This recipe makes approximately 7oz of butter. You will need an 8 oz glass jar, or two, 4 oz glass jars. Weigh all of the ingredients and have them ready prior to making.

Melt the following ingredients using the stovetop method:

- 1 oz beeswax
- 2 oz coconut oil
- 2 oz sweet almond oil or jojoba
- 2 oz cocoa butter

Note: The order of adding ingredients should be beeswax, coconut oil, cocoa butter, and sweet almond oil. You may add shea butter, if desired, by using 1 oz cocoa butter and 1 oz shea butter to make 2 oz butter. If you use shea butter, add this last to the pot. If you choose to add essential oils for extra benefits, you will add these last once the ingredients have melted and mixed. Pour in the jars, cover and allow to cool.

Subtle Shea Soft Butter

Use this recipe when you desire more of a lotion/creamy consistency. It is subtle in its natural aroma, but with a powerful impact on your skin. You can use unscented or add essential oils in the end, if desired.

This recipe yields about 8.8 oz (250 g) of finished product. The product has a silky and smooth texture which makes it ideal for application on the body with massage or as a light skin soother.

- 6.25 oz shea butter
- 4 oz jojoba oil
- 2 oz virgin coconut oil

Using the stove top method (with pyrex or double boiler):

- On low-medium heat, add all ingredients in the double boiler except your essential oils
- Slowly and continuously stir with a wooden spatula until melted
- Once melted, turn off the flame and let cool for 5 minutes
- Transfer to a glass bowl and let chill in the refrigerator for 10 minutes
- Take out and whip the lotion with a whisk or beater until you get the consistency you want
- Add essential oils (optional)
- Transfer butter into a mason jar or a pump bottle (easy for dispensing)

This homemade soft butter can be used for up to 8 months when stored properly in a cool and dry place away from sunlight.

Kombo Rescue Balm

Soothe aching joints and sore muscles with this pain relieving butter. Use approximately a 5% dilution of essential oils.

Makes two 4 oz glass jars, or four 2 oz glass jars

Ingredients:

- 3 oz almond oil, arnica infused oil, or another carrier oil
- 2 oz kombo butter (Pycnanthus angolensis)
- 1 oz beeswax (Cera flava)
- 1 ½ oz shea butter
- ½ oz cocoa butter
- 60 drops Juniper
- 60 drops Rosemary
- 50 drops Copaiba
- 30 drops Turmeric
- 25 drops Ginger
- 15 drops Orange

Using the stovetop method (pyrex or double boiler):

- Fill your pot about ¼ full with water, bring it to a gentle rolling boil.
- Melt your ingredients in this order: beeswax, cocoa butter, kombo butter, avocado oil, then shea butter and stir gently until it's melted.
- Remove pyrex from heat
- Add essential oils
- Pour butter into your jars. Let it cool for at least an hour before using it.

Kombo Pain Relieving Whipped Butter (large batch)

Makes approximately 5 Jars of 8oz (250 ml)

Ingredients:

- 250 g kombo butter
- 250 g shea butter
- 250 g cocoa butter
- 250 g virgin coconut oil
- 90 drops Rosemary
- 90 drops Juniper

- 20 drops Ginger
- 20 drops Turmeric
- 15 drops Orange

Using the stove top method (with pyrex or double boiler):

- Combine kombo butter, shea butter, cocoa butter and coconut oil and heat until melted
- Add essential oils and stir well until mixed thoroughly
- Set aside to cool and to let solidification begin (you can put in the refrigerator to speed up the cooling, be careful to not let it fully solidify or it will be harder to whip)
- Using a hand mixer or mixer stand–whip until you reach a nice consistency
- Keep in mind that it will stiffen up the more it cools and become less fluffy
- Put into containers

Pro tip: Scoop your mixture into a plastic bag, tie the top of the bag, cut a corner, and fill your containers. Much easier.

This makes an incredibly moisturizing body butter and skin rejuvenator. More than this, it's often used exclusively to soothe sore and aching muscles and joints (especially hands and shoulders) or to heal burns.

Shea, Cocoa, and Kombo Luxurious Body Butter

This recipe uses 'parts' sizing to make it easy for you to make however much you want. Play around and adjust as much as you'd like with this recipe. Do what you feel.

Ingredients:

- 2 parts shea butter
- 2 parts cocoa butter
- 1 part kombo butter
- Essential oil(s) as desired

Using the stove top method (with pyrex or double boiler):

Melt your shea butter, cocoa butter, and kombo butter down in a double boiler

Once melted and thoroughly mixed, place in the refrigerator until cool, and the top hardens slightly

Blend with a mixer on high speed for 3-4 minutes or however long it takes to get the consistency you'd like.

Store in an airtight container

Salves

Salves are solid combinations of oils and waxes. Beeswax and an infused oil make a good pair. They make very versatile products that can be used to treat many skin issues, sunburn, wounds, joint pain, respiratory issues.. The list goes on and on.

Since salves don't contain water–they last quite some time. The average shelf life is a year or so. You'll want to store your salves in a cool, dry, dark place; and maybe make smaller batches so you can use them in a season's time.

You can test the consistency by placing a spoon in the freezer before making your salve. When the beeswax melts, pour a little salve onto one of the cold spoons and place it back into the freezer for 1 to 2 minutes. This will simulate what the final consistency will be like. Once cooled, you can make adjustments by adding more oil (for a softer salve) or more beeswax (for a firmer salve).

> Pro tip: Depending on which base oils you use, you may consider adding in 1% vitamin E or 0.5% Rosemary CO2 extract. I add one of these antioxidants to my salves when using vegetable oils such as flax, rosehip seed, evening primrose, or borage.

Typically salves are applied to localized areas such as the neck and shoulders (for aches and pains), the chest (for clearing congestion, to support breathing during a cold), on cuts and abrasions or insect bites (such as our summer all-heal salve), and on dry, irritated areas of the skin (elbows, psoriasis patch).

A note on salves from Juliet Blankespoor:

"Covering a large expanse of the body in a salve is often not desirable. Herbs used for widespread joint inflammation or injury are typically applied as an herbal-infused oil via massage. Essential oils can be diluted directly into the herbal-infused oil as needed. Examples of herbal oils that are often massaged into the skin are: Saint John's wort, arnica (Arnica spp., Asteraceae), and poplar buds. The beeswax in salves helps to prolong its application on the skin, in addition to holding in moisture. This quality is especially helpful when tissues are very dry or irritated. Oils tend to rub off quicker than salves and require more frequent application. Salves are also solid and are more convenient to transport than oil, which has the potential to spill or leak." - Juliet Blankespoor

Are there contraindications for salves? Yes!

Moisture and heat are trapped by oils and salves, and they should not be used in weepy skin conditions, infections, and fresh burns.

Avoid the use of oils and salves on poison ivy rashes, weepy eczema, pimples, boils, fresh sunburn, and fungal and bacterial skin infections. Instead, use herbal compresses, soaks, baths or poultices, which are water-based applications. (Juliet Blankespoor: Herbal Infused Oils article).

Salve Recipes

Simple Salve

Use this recipe to make a custom salve of your choice. Makes 5 ounces.

Ingredients:

- 1 oz. beeswax
- 4 oz. herbal infused oil(s) of your choice (choose one or a combination)
- 10-20 drops essential oil of choice (optional)

Using the stove top method (with pyrex or double boiler):

- Place your beeswax in a double boiler and gently warm over low heat until the beeswax melts
- Add herbal oils and stir over low heat until well-mixed
- Remove from heat and add essential oil(s)
- **Quickly** pour warm mixture into prepared tins, glass jars, or lip balm tubes and allow to cool completely
- Label and store in a cool location for 1 to 3 years

Red Hot Recovery (Hot Cayenne Salve)

This warming salve will work wonders in soothing sore muscles and joints. This salve is beneficial when heat is indicated. Do not use over irritated skin, cuts and keep away from your mucous membranes and the face.

- Follow the simple salve recipe and use Cayenne infused oil, then add:
- 30 drops Copaiba
- 25 drops Frankincense
- 20 drops Peppermint essential oil
- Store and label

Comfrey Comfort

Bring comfort to sore, tense muscles and joints. Use for minor sprains, strains, bruises, and areas that need TLC.

- Follow the simple salve recipe and use Comfrey infused oil, then add:
- 40 drops Copaiba
- 20 drops Rosemary
- 20 drops Lavender
- Store and label

Calendula Lavender Salve

Wonderful for bug bites, burns and dry skin. Makes a 1 ounce jar of salve.

Ingredients:

- 1/8 cup calendula herbal oil
- 1/8 ounce beeswax
- 10 drops Lavender essential oil
- 10 drops German chamomile essential oil
- 5 drops Frankincense essential oil

Using the stove top method (with pyrex or double boiler):

- Measure calendula and weigh beeswax
- Put beeswax on low-medium heat and allow it to melt almost completely
- Add your herbal oil and stir occasionally until the beeswax melts.
- Remove the pot from the heat and wipe moisture off the bottom of the pan
- Add essential oils and stir with a fork until well combined
- Pour the salve mixture into a sterilized glass jar
- Put the lid on
- Allow the salve to sit and harden, untouched. Do not move until after it has hardened, or it will slosh around and become uneven.
- Once hardened, label and store

Vegan Balm with Carnauba

This balm recipe takes inspiration from the joys of spring gardening and the excitement of summer adventures. To create a salve that helps hydrate and soften dry or rough skin, we combine soothing calendula herbal oil, lavender essential oil, and Roman chamomile essential oil with rich cocoa butter.

Makes a great massage balm if you desire a base that is thicker and allows for more grip. A little goes a long way!

Ingredients:

- 33g (3 Tbsp.) organic Calendula herbal oil
- 40g cocoa butter
- 9g carnauba wax
- 1/4 tsp. vitamin E oil
- 12 drops Lavender essential oil
- 8 drops Roman Chamomile essential oil
- 10 drops Frankincense essential oil

Follow the simple salve recipe, using carnauba wax.

Using Essential Oils with Care

Before we get into the super fun stuff, let's go over essential oil safety, precautions, and contraindications.

Storing Essential Oils

It is important to keep essential oils in a dark amber or cobalt blue glass bottle with an orifice reducer. Keep the lid on tight to reduce oxidation and limit exposure to heat and sunlight. Essential oils do not really have hard-set expiration dates. However, essential oils can oxidize over time, and gradually lose their therapeutic value and aromatic quality.

The lifespan of essential oils might vary tremendously from one botanical to the next, from one distillation to the next, and from one supplier to the next.

Factors that Can Impact the Shelf Life of Essential Oils:

- Composition of essential oils' natural chemical constituents
- The quality of the botanicals used
- The methods, conditions and care used during distillation
- The care in bottling, storage, and handling of the essential oil by your supplier and any suppliers they obtained the oil from
- The storage conditions of the oil once you have received it

* For more information on shelf life for specific essential oil families, see Chemistry Basics.

Essential Oil Safety

When we take medications, whether off the counter or by prescription, we receive instructions about dosages. With nature, however, we don't get this level of instruction. The instructions for dosages and dilutions we learn from either our ancestors, or from qualified professionals who have provided us with the resources. It is important to note that just because something is "natural" does not mean it qualifies it as safe. It is necessary to learn about the oils, uses and benefits and contraindications prior to using them.

Here are a few things to be aware of for essential oil safety:

Phototoxicity

Some essential oils can increase sensitivity to ultraviolet light when applied topically. Phototoxicity will be much stronger directly after application, and will gradually decrease over an eight to twelve-hour period. If higher than normal concentrations are used, it may take a longer time.

The most common oils that cause phototoxicity are the citruses—with bergamot oil being the most reactive. Some citruses are phototoxic if expressed, but not if distilled, like lemon and lime oil. The best way to combat phototoxicity is to use proper dilutions, avoid direct exposure to UV rays after application, and avoid the use of citrus oils if exposure will occur after treatment. *"Recommend that the client stay out of the sun or sun tanning booth for at least twenty-four hours after treatment if photosensitizing essential oils were applied to the skin."*-naha.org

The best treatment for skin irritation from essential oils is to wash the area gently with soap and water, so you can remove any lingering traces of the phototoxic oil.

Then apply a plain, unblended fatty oil such as coconut, Aloe Vera gel, or hydrosol to help calm the area and reduce the damage. Avoid contact with eyes and mucous membranes.

Common Phototoxic Essential oils:

- Bergamot * *(Citrus bergamia)*
- Angelica *(Angelica archangelica)*
- Cumin *(Cuminum cyminum)*
- Lime (cold pressed) *(Citrus medica)*
- Tangerine (cold pressed)
- Yuzu *(Citrus juno)*
- Bitter orange (cold pressed) *(Citrus aurantium)*
- Grapefruit- Distilled or expressed (low risk) *(Citrus paradisi)*
- Lemon (cold pressed)

Non-phototoxic citrus oils:

- Bergamot: Bergapteneless (FCF: Furanocoumarin Free) *(Citrus bergamia)*
- Distilled lemon *(Citrus limon)*
- Distilled lime *(Citrus medica)*
- Mandarin – Tangerine *(Citrus reticulata)*
- Sweet orange *(Citrus sinensis)*
- Expressed tangerine *(Citrus reticulata)*
- Yuzu oil (expressed or distilled) *(Citrus juno)*

Skin Sensitization

Skin or dermal sensitization refers to an allergic reaction that occurs upon initial exposure to a substance, but may be barely noticeable, if at all.

With repeated exposure to the same material, or to something similar where there is cross-sensitization, it can eventually induce a severe inflammatory reaction ignited by the cells of the immune system (T-lymphocytes). The reaction will appear red, blotchy, and irritated—and can be quite painful.

The thing with dermal sensitization is that once it occurs with a specific essential oil–that person will most likely have prolonged sensitivity for many years or their entire life. Sensitization is unpredictable, as some people will be sensitive to a potential allergen and some will not. The best way to prevent sensitization is to avoid known dermal sensitizers and avoid applying the same essential oils every day for lengthy periods of time.

Dermal Irritants

Dermal irritants, on the other hand, will cause an immediate inflammatory reaction when applied to the skin. No, it's not a "detox". It can show up as redness or blotches and the severity will depend on the concentration of the oil that was used.

Do not use dermal irritants on:

- Anyone with inflammatory or allergic skin conditions
- Open or damaged skin
- A client that has sensitive skin. If you're not sure, do a patch test first.

DO NOT GET ESSENTIAL OILS INTO THE EYES. If an essential oil gets into the eye–don't rub it. Soak a cotton ball with milk or vegetable oil and wipe over the area affected. In severe instances–flood the eye area with lukewarm water for fifteen minutes.

Pregnancy

According to IFPA (International Federation of Professional Aromatherapists), the following essential oils (when properly diluted) appear to be safe for use during pregnancy:

- Benzoin
- Bergamot
- Black pepper
- Chamomile (German & Roman)
- Clary sage
- Cypress, eucalyptus
- Frankincense
- Geranium
- Ginger
- Grapefruit
- Juniper
- Lavender
- Lemon
- Mandarin
- Marjoram (sweet)

- Neroli
- Petitgrain
- Rose
- Sandalwood
- Orange (sweet)
- Tea tree
- Ylang ylang

According to Tisserand and Balacs, the following essential oils should not be used during pregnancy:

- Wormwood
- Rue
- Oak moss
- Lavandula stoechas
- Camphor
- Parsley seed
- Sage
- Hyssop

You can find the complete list of essential oils to avoid throughout pregnancy, labor, and while breastfeeding at www.NAHA.org.

Chemistry Basics

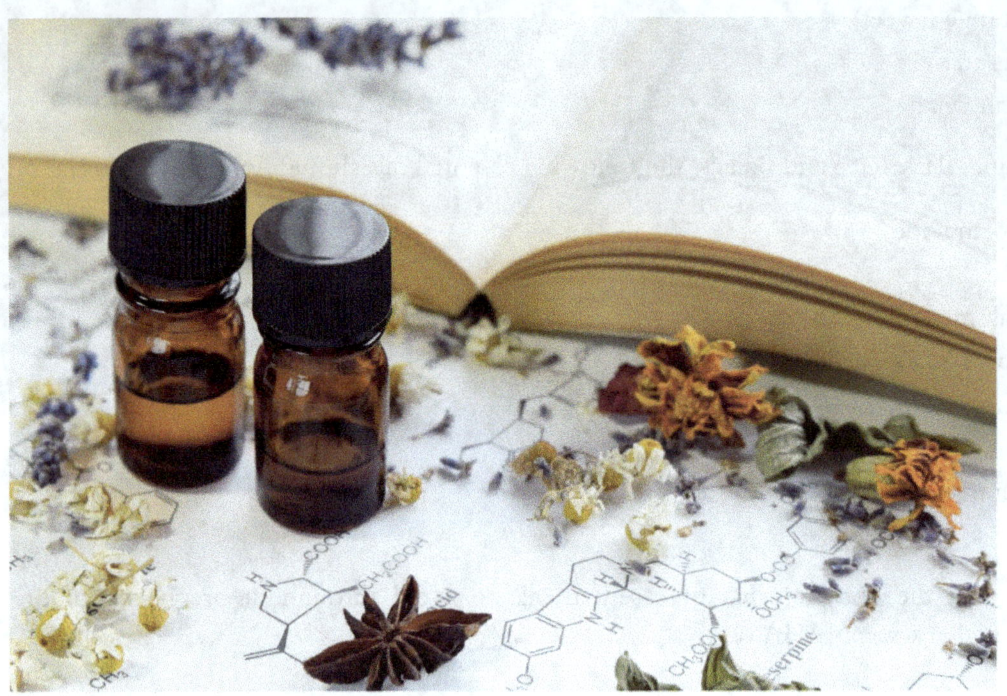

Taxonomy

Taxonomy is the science of classification, particularly vital when dealing with essential oils, which are from the plant kingdom. Distinguishing between different plant species by name is crucial due to the numerous variations of certain plants, such as lavender and chamomile, each possessing distinct properties.

In scientific notation, the first letter of the genus name is capitalized, and the species is in lowercase.

For example, here are 3 different species of eucalyptus:

- Eucalyptus globulus
- Eucalyptus radiata
- Eucalyptus citriodora

You will also notice that sometimes the Latin name contains an "x" in the middle. This indicates it is a cross or a hybrid.

For example, Lavender angustifolia + Spike Lavender = Lavandula x intermedia.

Chemotypes

Chemotypes are essential oils that have been extracted from the same genus and species, yet contain different chemical components.

How is this possible? Several factors contribute to this: wild plants cross pollinate, plants are grown at different elevations, growing conditions vary, climate plays a role, and other environmental factors are involved.

Because of the variations in chemical components, they usually have different therapeutic properties for aromatherapy practice, which is why this is important to be aware of.

For Example,

Lavender cultivated at higher altitudes may contain higher levels of certain chemical constituents, such as linalool and linalyl acetate.

- Rosmarinus officinalis ct. cineole: is high in the chemical component 1,8 cineole.
- Rosmarinus officinalis ct. verbenone: is high in the chemical components verbenone and pinene.

Chemistry

Essential oils are extremely complex and contain natural plant chemicals, also called constituents that are responsible for their healing properties. Some plants can contain up to 400 constituents! They work together synergistically to give the Essential Oil its power. They are not adulterated with additives of any kind. These natural elements provide numerous benefits for us. Let's look at a few…

Aldehydes

Aldehydes are a type of organic compound commonly found in essential oils. They are characterized by the presence of a carbonyl group (C=O) bonded to a hydrogen atom and a carbon atom. They are generally considered to have a sweet, fruity, and sometimes floral aroma.

Aldehydes are fresh smelling, uplifting, and soothing all at the same time. They are also anti-infectious, antifungal and anti-inflammatory. They help to ease the nervous system, can have a sedative effect, and are great for calming mental stress.

It is advisable to use a low dilution (1% or less), perform a patch test, and it may be best to avoid using them in the bath, even with a carrier, as they can cause skin irritation.

Examples of oils containing Aldehydes:

- Lemongrass (cymbopogan citrates)
- May Chang (Litsea cubeba)
- Lemon Verbena (Lippia citriodora)

- Lemon Eucalyptus (Eucalyptus citriodora)
- Melissa (Melissa officinalis)

Shelf life: 2-6 years

Alcohols

Essential oils contain another class of organic compounds known as alcohols, which typically have a mild, floral or woody aroma. In essential oil chemistry, alcohols are highly valued for their antimicrobial and anti-inflammatory properties.

Alcohols are often beneficial in skincare products, such as toners, as they can have a soothing or invigorating effect.

(linalool can have a sedative effect)

Examples of oils containing Alcohols:

- Tea Tree (Melaleuca alternifolia)
- Bergamot (Citrus bergamia)
- Peppermint (Mentha piperita)
- Palmarosa (Cymbopogon martinil)
- Geranium (Pelargonium graveolens)

Shelf life: 2-6 years

Esters

Esters are organic compounds that have an oxygen atom double-bonded to a carbon atom and also a carbon-oxygen bond. Esters have gained a reputation for their fruity, floral, and sometimes spicy aroma, making them a popular choice in perfumery for their pleasant and uplifting scents.

Aromatherapists highly value esters for their calming and soothing properties, frequently employing them to ease stress and anxiety. They also have mild analgesic and antispasmodic properties, which make them useful for treating muscle pain and cramps.

They have a relaxing effect on the CNS and are frequently utilized in nervous system tonics. They are carminative (help relieve gas), anti-inflammatory, and are soothing to dermal inflammations–which helps with scar healing.

Esters love the skin and are great for people who are stressed and hypertensive.

Examples of oils containing Esters:

- Lavender (Lavandula angustifolia)
- Roman Chamomiles ((Matricaria recutita and Chamaemelum nobile)
- Clary Sage (Salvia sclarea)
- Ylang Ylang (Cananga odorata)
- Geranium (Pelargonium graveolens)
- Petitgrain (Citrus aurantium amara)

Shelf life: 2-3 years

Ethers

Ethers possess a unique structure due to the presence of an oxygen atom bonded to two carbon atoms, which allows them to have a wide range of properties and uses.

Ethers promote healthy digestion, are mentally stimulating, respiratory stimulating, and have anti-inflammatory and antispasmodic effects that can be used to treat neuromuscular disorders. For individuals who are feeling weak or depressed, they can provide stimulation and promote a feeling of calm and tranquility.

Important to note: Ethers can easily irritate the skin, so use these in low doses (less than 1%) and for short periods. DO NOT USE long term.

Examples of oils containing Ethers:

- Basil (Ocimum basilicum)
- Anise (Illicium verum)
- Fennel (Foeniculum vulgare dulce)
- Nutmeg (Myristica fragrans)

Shelf life: 2-3 years

Ketones

Ketones are characterized by the presence of a carbonyl group (C=O) bonded to two carbon atoms. Ketones have a distinctive, sharp, and often medicinal aroma, and are often used for respiratory support. They help with infections in the respiratory tract and are strong mucolytics and expectorants.

They also have antifungal, antiviral, and analgesic properties–and stimulate the circulatory system. Ketones can also help with wound healing and tissue regeneration.

AVOID INTERNAL USE. It is important to use ketones with caution, as they can be toxic in high concentrations. Pregnant women and individuals with certain medical conditions, such as epilepsy or liver disease, should avoid using ketones altogether.

Examples of oils containing Ketones:

- Rosemary (Rosmarinus officinalis)
- Peppermint (Mentha piperita)
- Spike Lavender (Lavandula latifolia)
- Camphor (Cinnamomum camphora)
- Turmeric (Curcuma longa)

Shelf life: 2-3 years

Phenols

The presence of a hydroxyl group (-OH) directly attached to an aromatic ring gives phenols their special qualities and a powerful, distinguishable fragrance.

Phenols have a reputation for their powerful antimicrobial and antiseptic properties, and are often used in natural cleaning products and disinfectants.In aromatherapy, phenols are appreciated for their stimulating and invigorating properties, believed to enhance mental clarity and focus.

Phenols are chemically "hot" and are dermal irritants. Always use low dilutions (1% or under), carry out a patch test, and DO NOT use in the bath even with a carrier as they can severely irritate the skin.

Caution: Phenol compounds found in Essential Oils have been found to be potential liver toxins when taken internally in high doses or over lengthy periods of time. Use in low dilutions, and always with a carrier oil.

Examples of oils containing Phenols:

- Clove bud (Syzygium aromaticum)
- Cinnamon (Cinnamomum zeylanicum)
- Thyme (Thymus vulgaris)
- Basil (Ocimum basilicum)
- Oregano (Origanum vulgare)

Shelf life: 2-3 years

Monoterpenes

Monoterpenes are distinguished by their structure, which consists of two isoprene units that combine to create a molecule with ten carbon atoms. They are well known for their uplifting and stimulating effects, and are often used in aromatherapy to promote mental clarity, energy, and positivity.

They serve as excellent tonics, providing stimulation, energy, antibacterial properties, and a rubefacient effect, while also acting as mild expectorants (e.g., pine needle). However, they may dry out the skin and mucous membranes.

Oils high in monoterpenes, such as citrus oils oxidize quicker than other oils.

Fun Fact: Adding oils rich in monoterpenes into blends enhances transdermal penetration.

Examples of oils containing monoterpenes:

- Citrus oils such as Grapefruit (Citrus paradisi)
- Orange (Citrus sinensis)
- Lemon (Citrus limonum)
- Bergamot (Citrus bergamia)
- Black pepper (Piper nigrum)
- Pine (Pinus Sylvestris)
- Juniper (Juniperus communis)

Shelf life: 1-2 years

Sesquiterpenes

Sesquiterpenes form when three isoprene units combine to create a 15-carbon molecule. These organic compounds have very diverse therapeutic properties: they are anti-inflammatory, antiseptic, antibacterial, antispasmodic, sedating, pacifying, soothing, and calming to the nervous system.

These molecules tend to be heavier, often serving as middle to base notes with a long-lasting aroma due to decreased volatility (slower evaporation).

Examples of oils containing Sesquiterpenes:

- Balsam Copaiba(Copaifera officinalis)
- Cedarwood (Cedrus atlantica)
- Myrrh (Commiphora myrrha)
- German chamomile (Matricaria chamomilla)
- Ginger (Zingiber officinale)
- Lavender (Lavandula angustifolia)
- Patchouli (Pogostemon cablin)
- Vetiver (Vetiveria zizanioides)

Shelf life: 4-8 years

Basil *ocimum basilicum*

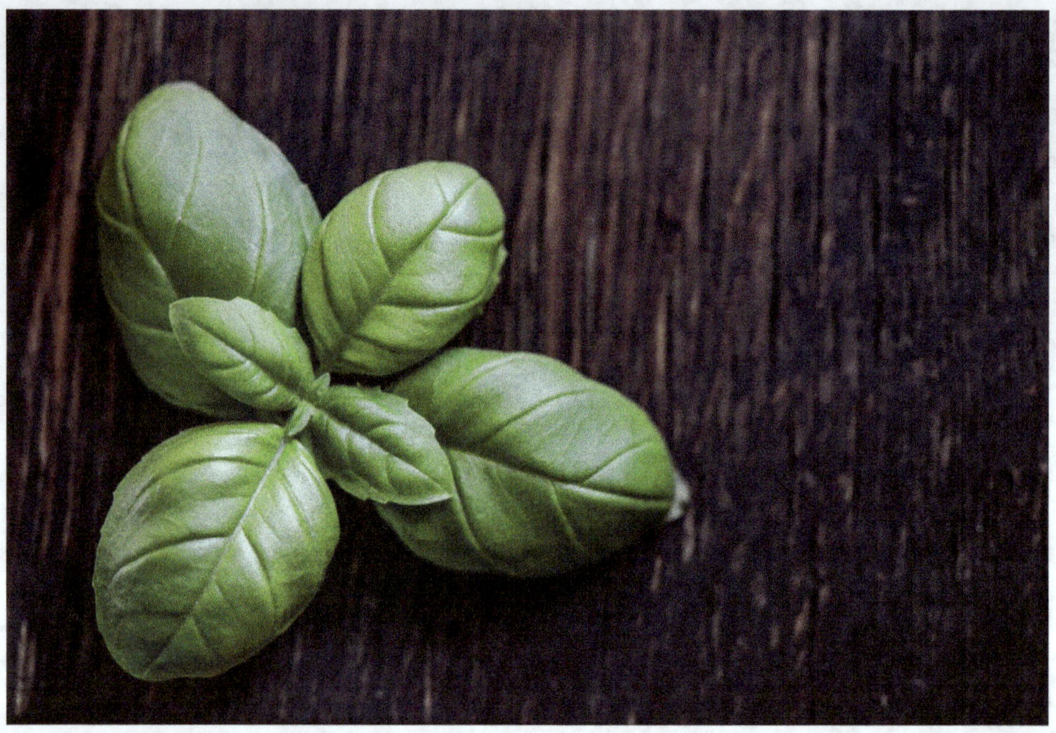

Warming, uplifting, energizing, awakening, clarifying and stimulating—that's sweet basil. If you or your client are feeling mentally fatigued, this herb brings a sense of calm and clarity like no other. It's sweet, spicy, and herbaceous with a tinge of licorice.

Background

Basil belongs to the lamiaceae family and its name comes from the Greek word that means royal or kingly. It's grown mostly in the USA, Vietnam, India, France, Italy and eastern Europe. We use the leaves of basil to extract its oil- and its most commonly extracted using steam distillation. Its major components are terpene alcohols—and it has an affinity for the nervous, immune, and musculoskeletal systems. Can grow up to 2 feet high.

Main Constituents: Methyl chavicol (estragole), Linalool, Eugenol, Cineole, Pinenine, Camphor

Country of origin: India, Egypt, Nepal, Hungary, France, USA, Italy, Spain, Vietnam

Extraction Method: Steam distillation

Part of Plant used: leaves

Therapeutics

Energizing, yet calming. Helps keep anxiety and stress at bay. Great for chest infections and digestive issues.

Physical:

- Nervous system tonic- restorative
- Muscular aches and pains
- Circulation
- Antispasmodic- muscular, menstrual cramps
- Digestive Tonic- indigestion, stomachaches, constipation
- Immune tonic- chest infections, colds and flu

Emotional:

- Intellectual Fatigue & Burnout
- Melancholic Depression
- Anxiety
- Nervous Tension
- Mental Stimulation- motivates and sharpens the mind
- Protection, Vulnerability
- Revitalizes and awakens the spirit

Blends well with

Rosemary, Lavender, Peppermint, Bergamot, Orange, lime, Eucalyptus, Grapefruit.

Bodyworker Applications

Tension Headache: 4 drops Basil + 4 drops Lavender + 5 drops Frankincense Oil + 2 drops Roman Chamomile + 1 oz. Carrier Oil.

Invigorating Massage Oil: Refresh tired muscles and invigorate the body and mind.

2 oz carrier oil + 7 drops basil + 6 drops Bergamot + 2 drops Eucalyptus Globulus + 2 drops Lavender + 3 drops Peppermint

Safety

Avoid during pregnancy. May be sensitizing, use well diluted. Maximum dilution of 3.3% for topical applications. External use only.

Bergamot *citrus bergamia*

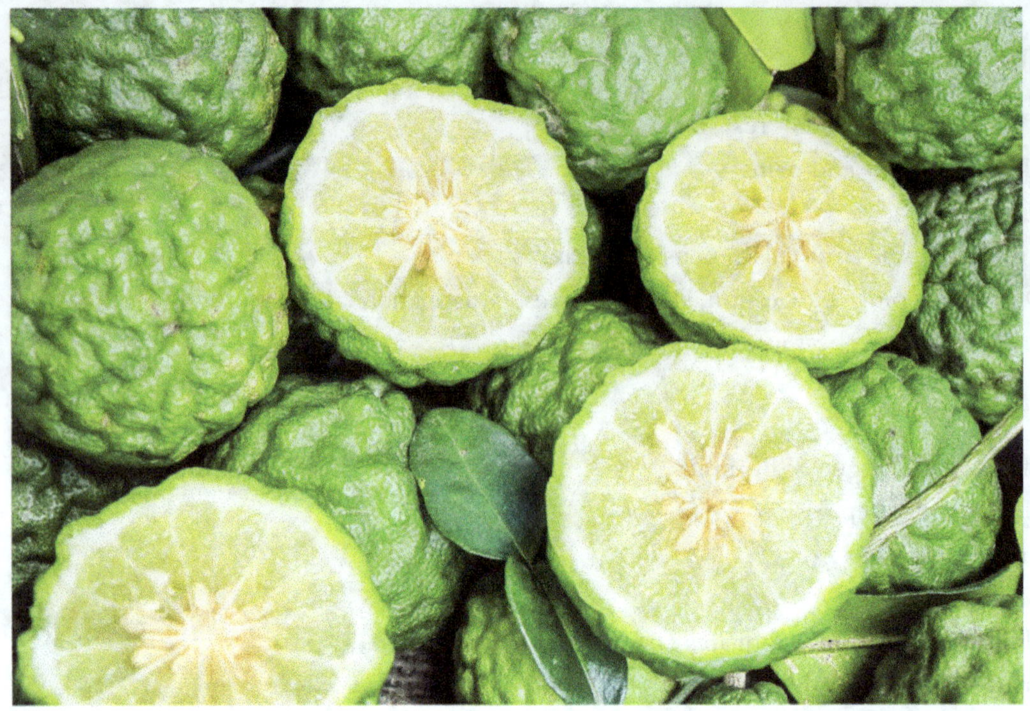

Often called "sunshine in a bottle," bergamot is playful, uplifting, and invigorating! Bergamot will brighten your day, while simultaneously soothing the senses.

Background

Bergamot received its name from the Italian city of Bergamo, where it was originally cultivated and sold. The essential oil is extracted through cold pressing the peel of the fruit; and it was one of the ingredients in the first "eau de cologne" formulas. Genetic research indicates that bergamot orange is likely a hybrid of lemon and bitter orange. It's famously associated with Earl Grey tea–and is used to compliment the taste in many black tea blends. Used as a primary ingredient in many high end perfumes, it is an all-time favorite essential oil.

Main Constituents: Up to 60 percent esters, (linalyl acetate), monoterpenes (d-limonene, pinene), furanocoumarin (5 to 10% bergaptene)

Country of origin: Italy

Extraction Method: Expression, steam distillation

Part of Plant used: peel of the fruit

Therapeutics

Brightens mood and uplifts spirits. Aids in alleviating anxiety, stimulates metabolism and is beneficial for hormonal balance.

Physical:

- Stimulates Metabolism
- Reduces Sluggishness
- Skin toning and Detoxifying
- Stress-related digestive problems
- PMS/Menopause hormonal imbalance
- Nervine

Emotional:

- Anxiety- one of the most studied essential oils
- Relaxant and sedative
- Balancing
- Lifts the spirits-depression, sadness
- Unreleased tension and frustration (pent-up feelings)- helps us to "just relax and let go"
- Mood Swings
- Mental clarity
- Improve sleep quality - reducing restlessness and insomnia.

Blends well with

Lavender, Basil, Clary Sage, Cedarwood, Cypress, Frankincense, Geranium, Peppermint, Nutmeg, Rosemary, Sandalwood, Ho Wood, Yarrow, and all citrus oils such as orange and mandarin.

Bodyworker Applications

Stress Relief Massage Oil: 3 drops Cedarwood Atlas + 3 drops Orange Sweet Oil + 3 drops Lime Oil + 3drops Bergamot Oil + 2 drops Geranium + 1 oz. Carrier Oil.

Bergamot Smiles Inhaler

5 drops Bergamot + 5 drops Lavender + 5 drops Sweet Orange + Inhaler tube

Safety

Bergamot is highly photosensitizing. Do not use it before going into a sun tanning booth or the sun. Use at low concentrations.

A Case Study on Bergamot:

Bergamot (Citrus bergamia) Essential Oil Inhalation Improves Positive Feelings in the Waiting Room of a Mental Health Treatment Center: A Pilot Study

Bergamot essential oil (hereafter BEO) has a long industrial and medicinal history (Navarra et al., 2015). It is characterized by a high content of limonene, linalool, and linalyl acetate. Several clinical studies on aromatherapy with BEO, in combination with other essential oils, have shown promising results: anxiety and stress reduction, anti-depression, pain relief, and blood pressure and heart rate reduction. Further human studies with BEO inhalation alone have also shown significant effects on anxiety reduction (Watanabe et al., 2015), depression reduction (Watanabe et al., 2015), and blood pressure (Chang and Shen, 2011; Ni et al., 2013) and heart rate reduction (Chang and Shen, 2011; Ni et al., 2013). In addition, BEO has minimal side effects, if any (Navarra et al., 2015), suggesting BEO inhalation may have potential therapeutic benefits including improving overall mental health and anxiety.

Bergamot Mint *Mentha citrata*

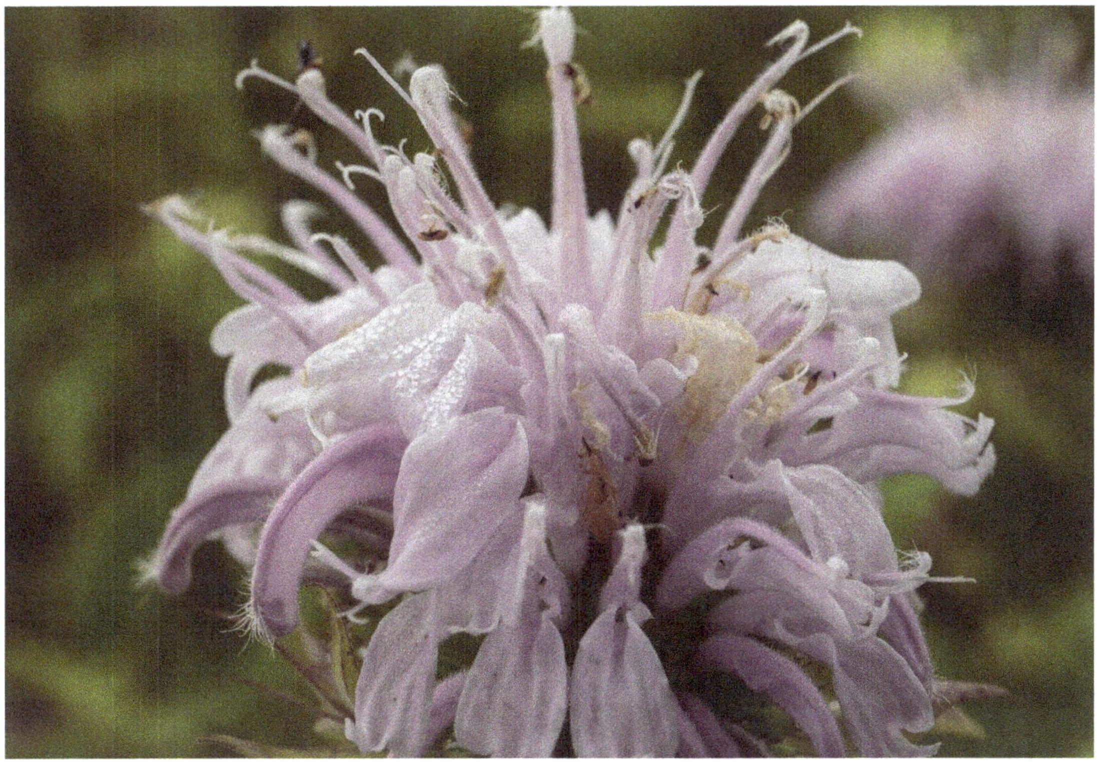

Imagine a gentle minty embrace with a hint of citrus and lavender—that's where the beauty of Bergamot Mint lies.

Bergamot mint is a favorite among pollinators, particularly bees and butterflies, hence its common name "bee balm." It is a herbaceous perennial plant native to North America. It is a member of the mint family (Lamiaceae) and shares a close relationship with other aromatic herbs like mint, oregano, and thyme. When you are hustling and bustling, Bergamot mint provides a serene escape to help you unwind and recover.

Background

Bergamot Mint It has a long history of use in folk medicine. Native American tribes traditionally used Bergamot Mint for various medicinal purposes. It is sometimes called "Oswego tea" because Native American tribes in the Oswego area of New York brewed tea from its leaves. The infusion from the leaves was used to treat ailments such as colds, fevers, sore throats, and digestive issues. The plant was also used topically as a poultice or salve to soothe skin irritations, insect bites, and minor wounds. Many people find its aroma rather intriguing with its soft hint of mint, citrus, and herbs.

Main Constituents: Linalool, linalyl acetate

Country of origin: North America

Extraction Method: Steam distillation

Part of Plant used: leaves

Therapeutics

Bergamot Mint Essential Oil is a delightful oil to work with and has a composition that is somewhat similar to that of Lavender Essential Oil, which makes it a lovely synergistic complement or substitute for lavender in particular blends.

Aromatically, Bergamot Mint essential oil has a fresh, citrusy aroma with minty undertones. It is often used in aromatherapy to uplift the mood, reduce stress, and promote relaxation. Because of its antiseptic and anti-inflammatory properties, bergamot mint essential oil may be beneficial for treating acne, soothing skin irritations, and promoting overall skin health. It also offers respiratory support-clearing congestion, relieving respiratory symptoms, and breathing during colds, coughs, and sinusitis. Bergamot mint is high in two main chemical constituents - linalool and linalyl acetate, which are responsible for its calming and uplifting aroma that is relaxing, soothing, and restorative.

Physical:

- Carminative- help relieve digestive discomfort
- Anti-inflammatory
- Antimicrobial
- Antispasmodic
- Skincare- anti-inflammatory, acne, irritations
- Cooling
- Respiratory support- decongestant
- Sore muscles

Emotional:

- Antianxiety
- Optimism
- Grounding
- Calming
- Stress

Blends well with

Lavender, Geranium, Palmarosa, Clary Sage, Bergamot, Orange, Mandarin, Ylang Ylang, Vetiver, Yarrow, and Cedarwood.

Bodyworker Applications

Abdominal Massage oil - Relieve tension and soothe digestive discomforts.

9 drops of Bergamot Mint + 4 drops Vetiver Oil + 3 drops Lavender Oil

2 drops of Mandarin + 1 oz Castor oil (or 50% castor oil & 50% carrier of choice)

Everything's Gonna be Alright - Inhaler blend

5 drops Mandarin + 5 drops Bergamot Mint + 5 drops Lavender + Aromatherapy Inhaler

Blissful Balance Massage Oil

5 drops Bergamot mint + 2 drops Ylang Ylang + 4 drops Lavender + 4 drops Bergamot + 1 oz carrier oil

Safety

May cause slight skin irritation for those with sensitive skin.

Black Pepper *Piper nigrum*

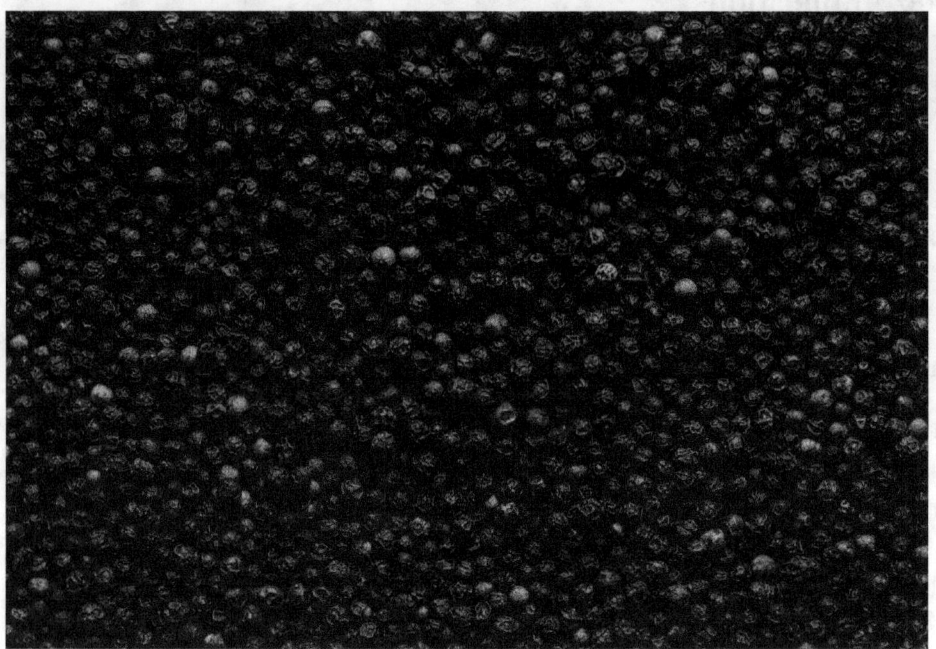

Warming, spicy, peppery and fresh, black pepper has an affinity for the muscles and joints. Enhance your blends with a little warmth and spice that stimulates movement and energy to areas that can benefit from the warmth and comfort. Inhale black pepper to stimulate your mind and wake you up in the mornings or any time you need to be revitalized!

Background

The essential oil is steam distilled from the sun-dried fruits of the peppercorn.

A clinical study published in Drug and Alcohol Dependence found that black pepper oil can suppress certain smoking withdrawal symptoms, including cravings for cigarettes.

Main Constituents:

β-Caryophyllene, d-3Carene

Country of origin: India, Sri Lanka, Madagascar,

Extraction Method: Steam distillation

Part of Plant used: Dried berries

Therapeutics

Energizing, yet calming. Helps keep anxiety and stress at bay. Great for chest infections and digestive issues.

Physical:

- Analgesic
- Expectorant
- Anti-inflammatory
- Antimicrobial
- Digestion - Bloating
- Circulation stimulant
- Stiff joints
- Reduces swelling/puffiness in the tissues

Emotional:

- Invigorating
- Fatigue
- Exhaustion
- Mental Stimulation - alertness and focus
- Smoking cessation
- Grounding

Blends well with

Bergamot, Clary Sage, Clove Bud, Ginger, Geranium, Grapefruit, Lavender, Juniper, Lime, Mandarin, Nutmeg, Rosemary, Yarrow, and Ylang-ylang.

Bodyworker Applications

Pepper Pacify Muscle gel: 4 drops Black Pepper Oil + 4 drops Bay Laurel Oil + 4 drops Lavender Oil + 1 oz Aloe Vera Gel + 3 ml Solubol (Dispersant)

Abdominal Massage blend: 2 drops Black Pepper + 1 drop Ginger + 2 drops Peppermint + 2 drops Sweet Orange + blend with 15 ml carrier oil

Work Wonders Recovery Oil: 4 drops Black Pepper + 4 drops Lavender + 4 drops Eucalyptus Globulus + 3 drops Rosemary + 1 oz carrier oil

Safety

Can cause skin irritation- use with care. Avoid during pregnancy and lactation.

Roman Chamomile *Chamaemelum nobile*

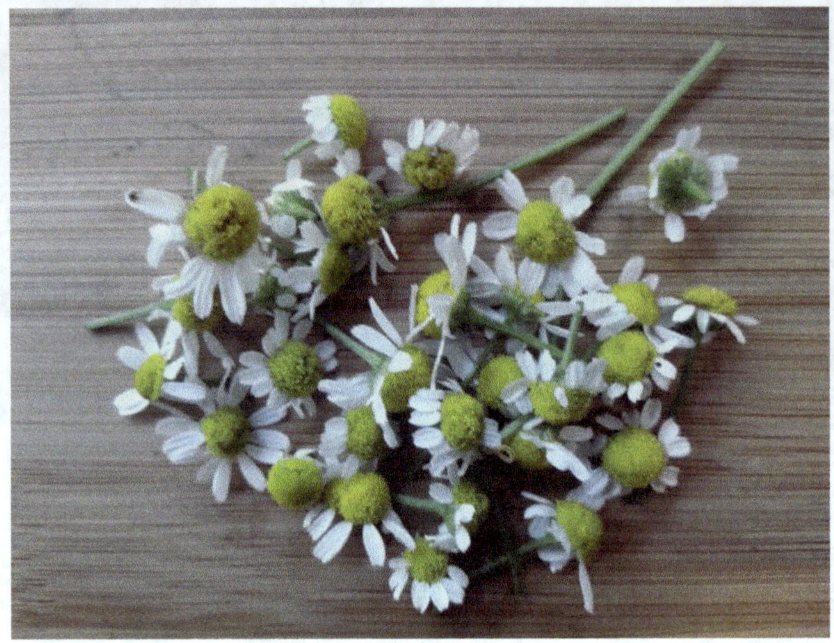

Roman Chamomile soothes your nervous system throughout the daily challenges. It will also tend to your skin if it's irritated and inflamed. If anxiety is affecting digestion, Chamomiles got your back!

Background

Chamomile is a low-growing plant with precious little daisy- like flowers. Throughout history, people have esteemed Roman chamomile for its medicinal properties. In Spanish, it is called "Manzanilla," which translates to "little apple," and the Greeks dubbed it "khamaimelon" or ground-apple because of its apple-like fragrance.

In Unani medicine, it was known as "roghan-e-baabunaa," valued for its anti-hysterical and antirheumatic properties. Even during the Second World War, it found use as a natural disinfectant, being 120 times more antiseptic than sea water. Pharmaceutical applications include its inclusion in antiseptic ointments and carminative preparations. Its anti-inflammatory properties make it effective against sunburn, while the cosmetic industry uses its oil in various products like soaps, perfumes, and hair care items. Chamomile's gentle nature makes it suitable even for the little ones, and people have relied on it as a gentle folk remedy for colic, restlessness, and the hyperactive child.

Main Constituents: Rich in esters ~ 80%

Country of origin: England, Italy, France, United States, South Africa, Hungary

Extraction Method: Steam distillation

Part of Plant used: Flowers

Therapeutics

Chamomile is a nerve tonic. These are herbs that the nourish, tone, rehabilitate and strengthen the nervous system. It is mild, yet extremely effective and can be used over a long period of time. Chamomile infusions are brewed from the flowers as a digestive aid and to soothe a "nervous upset stomach". It is a common choice as a sleep aid because it calms the nervous system and helps people wind down. Its anti-spasmodic and anti-inflammatory properties calm menstrual cramps and soothe inflamed skin and achy muscles. If you're feeling "tired but wired," Chamomile can help you get to the place of "rest and relax" so that your nervous system can recover.

Physical:

- Anti-spasmodic
- Analgesic-mild
- Anti-inflammatory
- Antimicrobial
- Digestion - indigestion, flatulence
- Skin- inflamed skin conditions (dermatitis, eczema, psoriasis, hives, acne)
- Slow healing wounds
- Muscle cramps
- Menstrual cramps

Emotional:

- Soothes the mind
- Calming
- Sedative
- Adrenal Fatigue
- Restlessness- feeling "tired but wired"
- Impulsiveness
- Irritability
- Nervous tension
- Anxiety

Blends well with

Lavender, Bergamot, Clary Sage, Orange, Mandarin, Geranium, Grapefruit, Lavender, Juniper, Lime, Lemongrass, Vetiver, Ho Wood, Frankincense, Yarrow, and Ylang-ylang.

Bodyworker Applications

Ahhh! My Nervous System Inhaler- Balance and tone the nervous system: 6 drops Roman Chamomile + 5 drops Lavender + 4 drops Bergamot + Aromatherapy Inhaler

Harmony Essence Inhaler- For depression and anxiety: 7 drops Roman Chamomile + 3 drops Geranium + 5 drops Grapefruit + Aromatherapy Inhaler

Dreamscape Massage Butter: 40 drops Lavender + 40 drops Roman Chamomile + 20 drops Mandarin + 15 drops Clary Sage + 1 batch ~ 7 oz of Skin Silk Butter. Make one large jar or divide into small jars. Add essential oils last.

Safety

No known safety issues. Patch test those who have hypersensitivities to ragweed, which is in the same family.

Himalayan Cedarwood *Cedrus deodara*

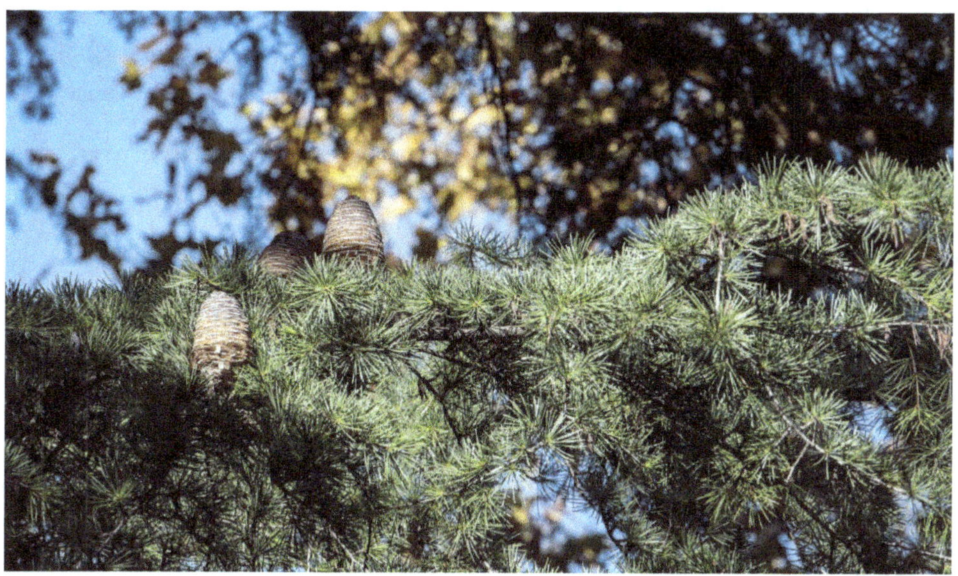

"It is not because things are difficult that we do not dare; it is because we do not dare that they are difficult. -Seneca

When you think about Cedarwood—think grounding, endurance, and strength. Traditional healers commonly employed this oil to improve mental clarity and promote balance. It is indicated when life gets chaotic or there are conflicting emotions and you need to get grounded to process your thoughts to take the next step or just meditate and reflect on the situation. It helps us to breathe when we feel constricted, whether physically or emotionally, and clears the respiratory tract. A classic for promoting stress relief due to its warm, comforting, and sedative properties.

Its aroma is woodsy, with a dry, smoky, balsamic undertone. The cedars have an inherent ability as a base note to hold a flighty blend together. It's one of those oils that I love to blend or diffuse year-round as needed. Although every plant has its own unique aromatic profile and chemical makeup, the cedarwood oils share similar properties.

Background

A tall evergreen tree up to 50 m high. It grows extensively on the slopes of the Himalayas in northern India, Pakistan and Afghanistan. The word cedar comes from the Arabic Kedron meaning "power".

Cedar oil has also been widely used in Eastern medicine and various cultures to address ailments ranging from minor physical discomforts, including coughs and colds, to more severe illnesses.

Atlas Cedarwood:

Related C. deodara. A pyramid-shaped evergreen conifer is native to the Atlas Mountains of Algeria and Morocco. The ancient Egyptians used it for embalming, cosmetics and perfumery. Not to be confused with the North American 'Red Cedar' tree in the cypress family.

A study using Cedrus atlantica essential oil used in an aromatherapy massage blend for the treatment of Alopecia areata—a disorder in which the hair falls out in patches producing baldness. The group using the massage blend containing Atlas cedarwood showed a significant improvement of 44%. Hay IC, Jamieson M, Ormerod AD. Randomized trial of aromatherapy—successful treatment of Alopecia areata.

(Archives of Dermatology, 1998; 134(11): 1349-1352. Cited in the Aromatherapy Database, By Bob Harris, Essential Oil Resource Consultants, UK, 2000.)

Atlas Cedarwood is often used for hair and scalp care and the treatment of seborrheic dermatitis with dandruff,

Atlas cedarwood is now on the IUCN Red List of Threatened Species as endangered. It is now widely cultivated in Europe. Much of the Atlas cedarwood oil produced nowadays is from plantation trees.

Main Constituents: β-Himachalene, α-Himachalene

Country of origin: India, Nepal

Extraction Method: Steam Distilled

Part of Plant used: Wood

Therapeutics

Grounding and calming. Fortifies the body's systems- strength and power—while helping to ease stress.

Physical:

- Stimulant- circulatory and lymphatic system
- Expectorant - Mucolytic
- Cold damp conditions
- Bronchitis - coughing
- Analgesic
- Astringent
- Diuretic
- Antiviral
- Antifungal
- Aphrodisiac
- Alopecia areata
- Lymphatic - decongestant, encourages lymphatic drainage

- Cellulite reducing- counteracts water and lipid retention
- Improves oily skin, acne
- Dandruff
- Dermatitis-Eczema
- Skin- regulates sebum production

Emotional:

- Sedative (nervous)
- Grounding
- Emotional equilibrium- stressful transitions
- Calms the Shen- anxiety, restlessness
- Meditation, reflection - helps us to "press pause" with the non-stop lifestyle or when life gets chaotic.
- Worry, stress that inhibit relaxation
- Stress and nervous tension that lead to fatigue and burnout

Blends well with

Juniper, Lavender, Rosemary, Cypress, Grapefruit, Bergamot, Lime, Lemon, Orange

Bodyworker Applications

Soothing Muscle Comfort blend: 5 drops Cedarwood + 4 drops Cypress + 4 drops Rosemary + 2 drops Sweet Orange + 1 oz carrier oil

Your Mind at Ease Inhaler Recipe

8 drops Bergamot + 6 drops Cedarwood + 4 drops Lavender + 1 drops Vetiver

Oh Yeah! Body Scrub

2 drops Cedarwood + 2 drops Sweet Orange + ½ Cup Raw Cane Sugar + ¼ cup carrier oil

Safety

Non-toxic, non-irritant and non-sensitizing. Avoid use during pregnancy and with children under 6 years. Do not take cedarwood essential oil internally.

Clary Sage *salvia sclarea*

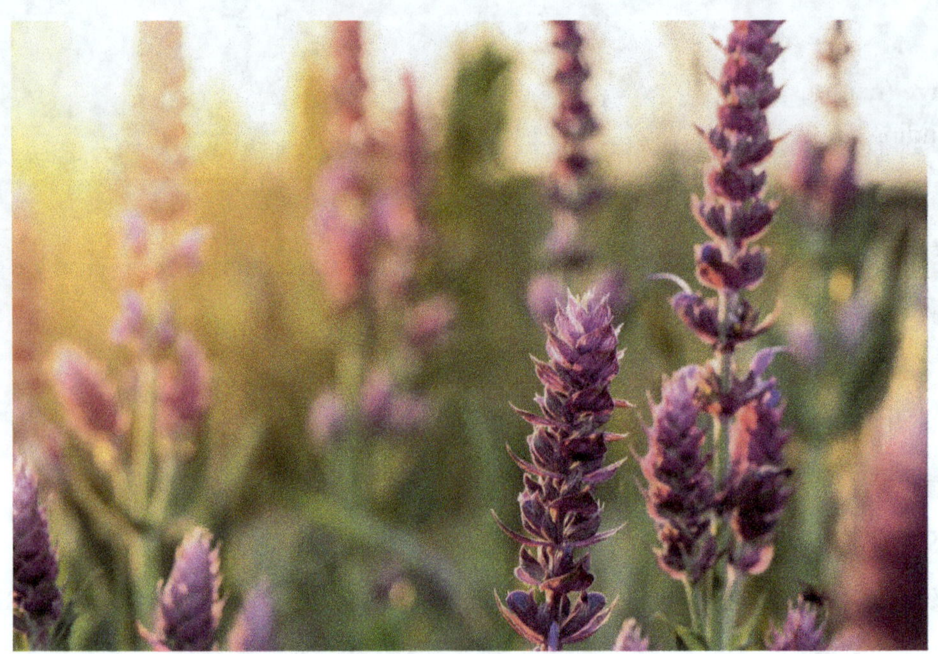

"Perhaps it was the flowers that made me a painter" - Monet

'Good for everything'.. that's the legacy of Clary Sage. This highly aromatic plant is deeply calming while igniting a state of euphoria. Research indicates it is a powerful and transformational oil for the treatment of depression. The distinct musky, nutty, and pungent aroma of Clary Sage finds extensive use in perfumery.

Background

A member of the plant family, Labiatae (Lamiaceae), Clary Sage is originally native to southern Europe. The whole plant is highly aromatic and the flowering stalks are cut in the summer for essential oil extraction.

Main Constituents: Esters (especially linalyl acetate, 75%)

Country of origin: France, Spain, Bulgaria, Italy, USA, England, Morocco, Germany, South Africa, Russia

Extraction Method: Steam distillation

Part of Plant used: Flowering tops

Therapeutics

Deeply calming, and euphoric for a mental-emotional uplift. As a nervine, Clary sage supports us when chronic stress and mental fatigue leads to debility. It balances us when we feel "tired but wired". When our bodies are unable to find balance between stimulation and relaxation, it aids us in resting and recovering. It also helps eliminate the spread of bacteria—making it a great ingredient in natural deodorant.

Physical:

- Powerful Muscle Relaxant: Helps with aches and pains, arthritis and rheumatism.
- Antispasmodic
- cools skin inflammations
- PMS/Menopause discomfort- stiffness, muscle cramps
- Has an affinity for the reproductive and endocrine systems
- Nerve tonic-sedative
- Anti-inflammatory
- Pain relieving

Emotional:

- Calming- anxiety and stress
- Euphoric
- Balancing
- Anger
- Depression
- Racing thoughts- calms the mind
- Disconnection

Blends well with

Bergamot, Chamomile, Lavender, Geranium, Bergamot, orange and other citrus, cedarwood, Frankincense Fennel, Frankincense, Vetiver, Yarrow, and Ylang Ylang.

Bodyworker Applications

A Woman's Balance Bath Soak: 3 drops Clary Sage + 2 drops Geranium + 3 drops Lavender + 2 drops Bergamot + 1 Cup Epsom salt + 1 tbsp. Carrier oil + 1 tbsp. Castile soap (optional)

Sleep Peacefully - a beautiful oil blend that can be used in roll on bottles, as a massage oil (add to 1 tsp. Carrier oil), or for inhalation on diffusing.

3 drops Clary Sage + 2 drops Lavender Oil + 2 drops Atlas Cedarwood

The Fidgeter

Clary Sage is great for clients who just can't lay still and shut their mind off! Combine clary sage with Lemongrass to calm the mind and will soothe the nervous system. Can be used in place of Lavender if looking for another option for calming, antispasmodic, etc.

Euphoric Elation Synergy- Makes 4 ml. Dilute with a carrier for a massage oil (1 - 2% dilution) use in a diffuser.

1 ml Clary Sage + 1 ml lavender + 1 ml Sweet Orange + .5 ml Ylang Ylang + 1 ml Bergamot

Safety

Non-toxic and non-irritant. Non- to mildly sensitizing. Consult your health care professional before using during pregnancy. Do not take clary sage essential oil internally. May cause drowsiness when used in high doses.

Copaiba Oleoresin *copaifera officinalis*

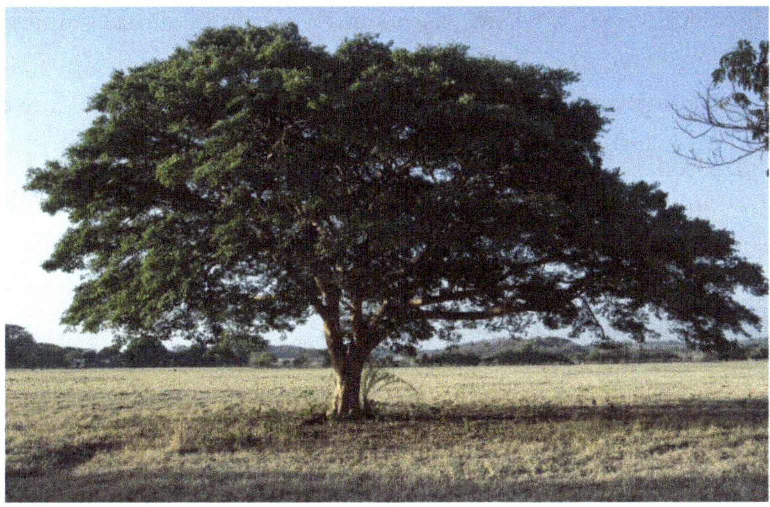

Copaiba is probably most well known for keeping wounds from being infected. It's a unique, gentle oil that comes from the Amazon. Copaiba essential oil and oleoresin contain large amounts of Beta-caryophyllene, a molecule that interacts with cannabinoid receptors in your skin. This causes skin cells to produce beta-endorphin, one of the happiness hormones.

It's got a light, woody, sweet and balsamic scent.

Background

Copaiba oleoresin is tapped from the Balsam of the Copaiba tree of the Amazon. Local populations in the Amazon have long regarded copaiba oil as being antiseptic and antibacterial and have relied on it to prevent wounds from getting infected. Copaiba makes a wonderful fixative, holding a blend together, without overpowering it.

Main Constituents: Sesquiterpenes

Country of origin: Brazil, amazon regions

Extraction Method: Tree tapping, Steam distillation

Part of Plant used: Oleoresin

Therapeutics

Great for wound healing. Warming, anti-inflammatory, euphoric, regenerative, gentle, and supports the respiratory system. The high concentration of sesquiterpenes in Copaiba Balsam gives it powerful anti-inflammatory properties and it also possesses anti-bacterial and antimicrobial effects.

Physical:

- Musculoskeletal: Anti-inflammatory, pain relieving, swollen inflamed joints, cooling.
- Respiratory System: Antiseptic, anti-catarrhal and expectorant for the respiratory tract (including bronchitis and sinusitis).
- Digestive system: Antiseptic, soothes gastric and other internal inflammations, stomach ulcers, sore throats and tonsillitis
- Urinary system: anti-inflammatory and antiseptic for the urinary tract (for cystitis, bladder, and kidney infections), bacterial infections

Skin: wound healing, soothing irritation and treating eczema, psoriasis and other chronic skin disease

Emotional:

- Nurturing, uplifting, warming, comforting, gentle
- Lightens the spirit with its delicate aroma of the rainforest
- Stress relief
- Antidepressant

Blends well with

Chamomile, Lavender, Geranium, Bergamot, Orange and other citrus, Cedarwood, Frankincense, Yarrow, and ylang ylang.

Bodyworker Applications

Nerve TLC - soothing nervine blend

5 drops of Roman Chamomile essential Oil + 3 drops Clary Sage essential oil + 5 drops of Copaiba Oleoresin + 1 oz st. John's wort Infused Oil

FlexFlow Massage Oil

6 drops Lemongrass essential oil + 3 drops Plai essential Oil + 3 drops Copaiba Oleoresin + 3 drops Turmeric essential Oil + 1 oz carrier oil

Soothing Low Scented Massage oil - ideal for sensitive individuals

3 drops of Copaiba Oleoresin + 2 drops of Lavender Oil + 1 oz of Sweet Almond or Apricot Oil

Safety

Non-irritating, non-sensitizing, non-toxic. No contraindications known.

Cypress *cupressus sempervirens*

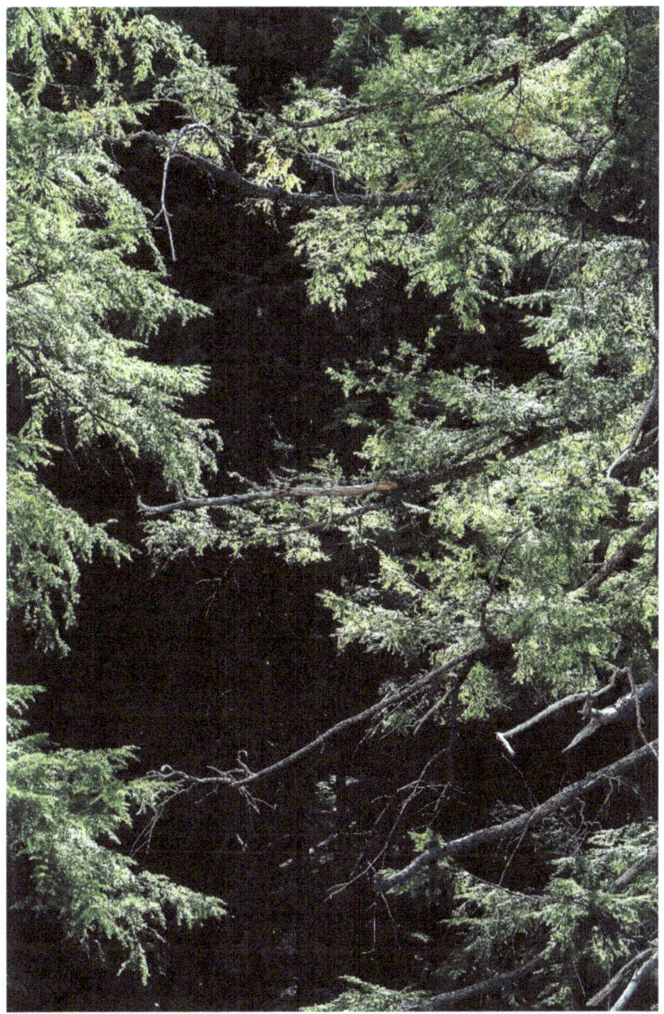

"You must do the thing you think you cannot do." - Eleanor Roosevelt

Cypress clears the air, expands the mind, and allows you to take a deep breath. This piney, smokey and refreshing tree releases its essential oils through its needles and branches via steam distillation. We love Cypress most for its healing powers on the respiratory and lymphatic systems.

Background

Native to the eastern Mediterranean, the name Sempervirens can be translated to "ever living".

A member of the Cupressus family of evergreen shrubs and trees, one of the oldest known plant families. The tree can grow between 40-60 feet and its leaves are dark green. Researchers have recorded some Cypress trees to be over 2,000 years old. The Mediterranean cypress earned the nickname "drama tree" due to its tendency to bend even with the slightest of breezes.

Main Constituents: Rich in monoterpenes (up to 45%)

Country of origin: France, Spain

Extraction Method: Steam distillation

Part of Plant used: Needles

Therapeutics

Helps circulate Qi and blood, expands the lungs, and clears the mind.

Physical:

- Circulates Qi and blood
- Congested lymphatic system
- Anti-Inflammatory
- Analgesic
- Vasodilator- used supporting vein health, helping with varicose veins
- Soothes the nervous system
- Gentle on the skin- astringent, oily skin
- Muscle Fatigue
- Contusion
- Menstrual issues-menorrhagia, dysmenorrhea, cramps

Emotional:

- Comforting- times of transition and mourning
- Stabilizing
- Promotes focus, creativity, and productivity
- Feelings of emotional "heaviness" or stagnation
- Supports and strengthens when there is stress related overwhelm- use with lavender

Blends well with

Bergamot, Lavender, Lemon, Chamomile, Cedarwood, Clary Sage, Frankincense, Grapefruit, Geranium, Ginger, Immortelle, Juniper, Orange, Rosemary, Pine and Petitgrain.

Bodyworker Applications

Love Your Skin Body Scrub:

5 drops Cypress + 7 drops Grapefruit + 3 drops Lavender or Palmarosa

1 cup Sea Salt + ½ cup Coconut Oil

Varicose Vein Soothe

15 drops cypress + 5 drops Lime + 10 drops Geranium 1 oz carrier oil

Gently apply to legs. Can be used twice per day, morning and evening, especially after a long day on your feet! Elevate your legs and relax.

Safety

Avoid prolonged exposure, particularly with allergy-sensitive individuals.

Eucalyptus *eucalyptus globulus*

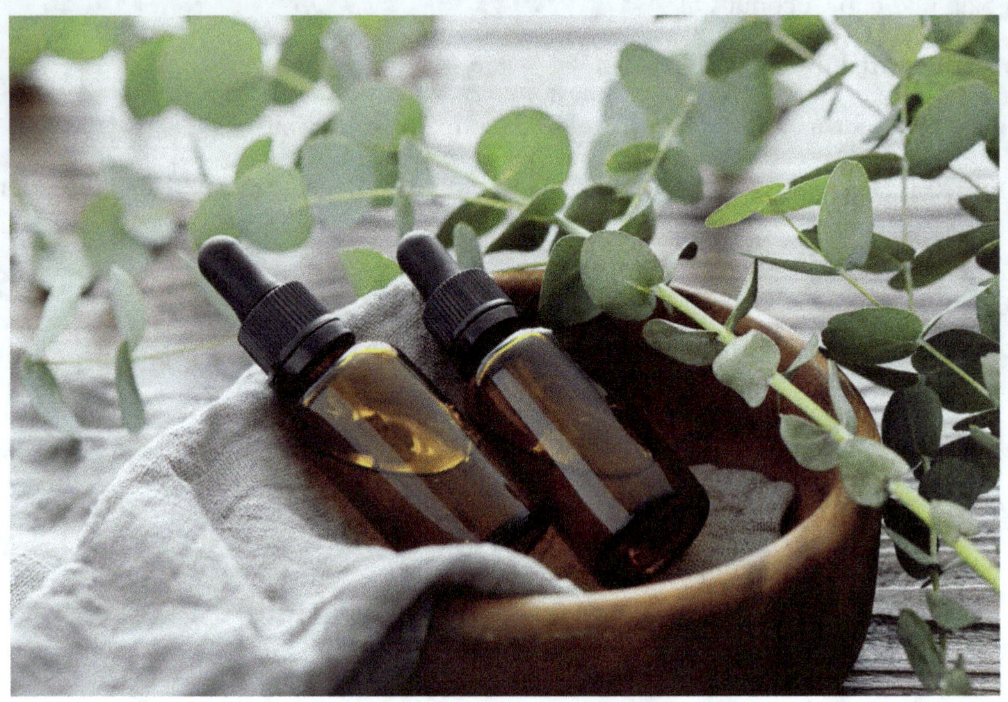

"If you have only one breath left, use it to say thank you."
- Pam Brown

"The fragrance of renewal." This incredibly clearing and powerful herb is a staple go-to for the common cold and congestion. Harvested from the leaves and twigs of the plant. Its aroma is crisp, green, and camphorous.

Background

Also called Blue Gum Eucalyptus–it is one of the most well-known varieties of eucalyptus. It can grow up to 300 feet tall and has round greenish silver leaves with white or cream-colored flowers.

The genus name Eucalyptus originates from Greek eucalyptos, meaning "well-covered," and describes its flowers, which, in bud, have a cup-like membrane that the flower sheds when it expands.

Main Constituents: 75% terpenes, cineole, sesquiterpenes and alcohols

Country of origin: Australia, China, Spain, Portugal

Extraction Method: Steam distillation

Part of Plant used: leaves

Great for a cold, and relieving sinus pressure. Deeply penetrating and revitalizing for the senses.

Therapeutics

Eucalyptus is most well-known for its therapeutic benefits for the respiratory system.

Physical:

- Lung Qi Tonic (TCM)-Opens the breath
- Analgesic - Muscular Aches And Pains
- Infectious disease: Antibacterial, antiviral, antiseptic
- Decongestant
- Expectorant
- Cooling
- Deodorizing
- Sinusitis
- Fever
- Rheumatism
- Respiratory infection
- Bronchitis

Emotional:

- Clears the mind and aids in concentration/clarity
- Mental Exhaustion
- "Clears the air"- negative feelings
- Invigorating- refreshing your space
- Stimulating
- "Room to breathe"- when feeling emotionally or physically constricted
- Emotional balance

Blends well with

Rosemary, Lemon, Bergamot, Black Pepper, Lime, Peppermint, Lavender, Cypress, Cedarwood and Lemongrass.

Bodyworker Applications

Deep Inhalations- To open up the sinuses and to release emotional constrictions and blockages.

Muscle Comfort- For Pain Relief & Stiffness

4 drops Eucalyptus Globulus + 4 drops Black Pepper + 3 drops Rosemary or Cypress + 3 drops Lavender + 1oz Carrier Oil

Safety

Caution with High blood pressure/epilepsy, may be an antidote to homeopathic remedies. Avoid during pregnancy, or while breastfeeding. Keep away from children. Radiata is preferred for children or the elderly.

Frankincense *boswellia carteri*

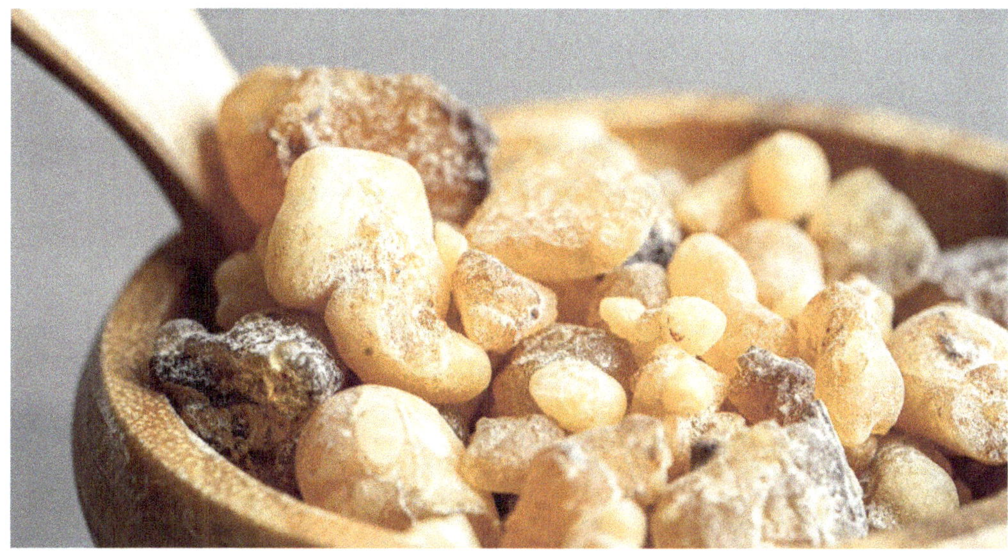

Frankincense is healing–for just about everything. Known as the one "true incense," its robust, sweet aroma brings ease and comfort to the senses. This resin has found wide usage in traditional medicines and perfumes.

Background

Native to Somalia, the crude gum of the tree undergoes distillation to extract the essential oil. Researchers have widely studied its medicinal actions and aromatherapeutic applications. The tree can grow up to 30 ft tall and thrives in dry, rocky climates. When the tree is pierced, it releases its aromatic resin which forms droplets known as 'tears' or 'pearls' as it hardens.

Main Constituents: Rich in esters and Monoterpenes

Country of origin: Somalia

Extraction Method: Hydro-distilled

Part of Plant used: resin

Therapeutics

Frankincense is unparalleled in inducing a meditative state. It is profoundly soothing, comforting, and uplifting.

Physical:

- Uplifting- inspires the mind
- Antibacterial
- Immune enhancer
- Anti-inflammatory
- Swollen joints- arthritis
- Expectorant
- Muscular Aches and Pains
- Would healer- inflamed skin conditions
- Scar tissue
- Dry or mature skin

Emotional:

- Promotes a meditative state of peace and calm
- Sedative
- Antidepressant- sense of worthlessness, self-destruction
- Nervine
- Carminative- anxiety, tension, fear
- Stills the mind-agitation, inability to focus

Blends well with

Bergamot, Clary sage, Atlas Cedarwood, Helichrysum, Geranium, Juniper, Lavender, Mandarin, Yarrow, and Ylang Ylang.

Bodyworker Applications

Soothing and Balancing Massage Blend:

1 oz carrier oil + 6 drops Frankincense + 4 drops Lavender + 2 drops Geranium

Joint Comfort: A warming blend to soothe arthritis and inflammation in the joints.

1 oz Carrier oil + 8 drops Frankincense, 3 drops Sweet Orange + 4 drops Ginger, 4 drops Turmeric

Grounding & meditation Diffuser Blend

Frankincense, Atlas Cedarwood, Helichrysum

Safety

Considered non-toxic, non-photosensitizing, and non-sensitizing.

Rose Geranium
pelargonium graveolens var roseum

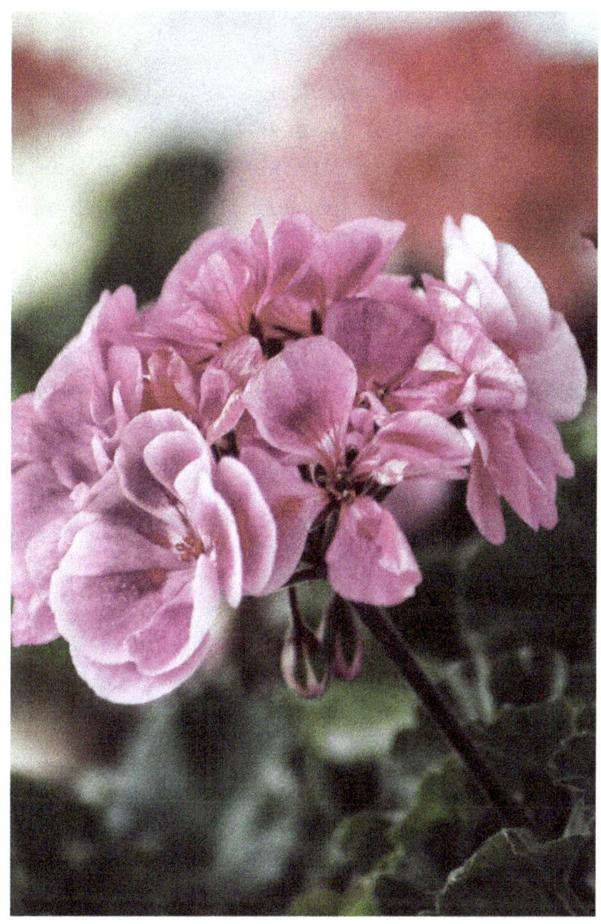

"Looking for and enjoying all beauty is a way to nourish the soul." - Matthew Fox

People used to go to great lengths to get their hands on Rose Geranium. Why? Geranium makes you feel beautiful. The fragrance is incredibly tempting, delightfully sweet, and absolutely captivating. It warms the heart, brings comfort to the soul, and ignites a thirst for life again!

Geranium's floral fragrance makes it a pleasure to use on its own or with other oils. In an unusual and enchanting way, it adapts to the blend. It brings balance when we feel off-balanced. It soothes us when our spirit needs soothing during emotional rigidity and distress. Geranium loves to shine with its astringent and skin-loving properties- reducing puffiness and balancing your skin's sebum production. Yes, Geranium makes you feel beautiful!

Extracted from the leaves via steam distillation.

Background

The name Geranium derives from the Greek word geranos or 'crane' because the seed pods resemble the shape of a crane's bill. It has been used widely in perfumery and soap manufacturing since the 19th century. There are more than 700 varieties of Geranium, however only about 10 provide the Essential Oil.

Rose Geranium belongs to the Pelargonium botanical family, a group also referred to as the "Fragrant Geraniums." It shares virtually all the same properties as geranium essential oil but is considered to be superior for the rosy floral note of its fragrance. If you do not have access to Rose Geranium essential oil, that's ok. Geranium essential oil and Rose Geranium essential oil are both derived from the Pelargonium graveolens plant species, but from different varieties. They have almost identical compositions and properties, making them equally beneficial in aromatherapeutic applications.

In the Victorian era, scented Geraniums were grown along the edges of pathways or placed pots indoors in the winter where women's wide crinoline skirts would brush past and release their pleasant scent.

Main Constituents: Rich in esters and alcohols

Country of origin: South Africa, Reunion Islands, Egypt, Madagascar, China, USA

Extraction Method: Steam distillation

Part of Plant used: Flowering tops

Therapeutics

The intoxicating aroma of Geranium brings comfort to the heart during occasional or ongoing stressful periods.

Physical:

- Cooling -Yin
- Skincare- balances sebum production, toning, healing
- Poor circulation- vasoconstrictor
- Edema
- Muscle spasms
- Inflammation-cooling heat
- Cellulite blends
- Stimulates the lymphatic system

Emotional:

- Emotional balance-harmonizing
- Mood swings and depression
- Hormone balancing - PMS, menopause
- Used in TCM to dissolve stagnation and promote Qi flow- Feeling "stuck"
- Chronic and acute anxiety- promotes strength and security
- Fatigue-agitation
- Nervous exhaustion- due to overwork
- Emotional numbness, disconnection- reconnect and "feel life"

Blends well with

Bergamot, Grapefruit, Lavender, Clary Sage, Orange, Peppermint, Frankincense, Jasmine, Rose, Ylang Ylang, Yarrow, Roman Chamomile and Eucalyptus.

Bodyworker Applications

Balancing and Uplifting Massage:

2 oz Carrier Oil + 8 drops Geranium + 6 drops Lavender + 5 drops Bergamot + 4 drops Grapefruit

Soothe the Skin Facial Oil:

2 drops Geranium + 3 drops Frankincense + 1 drop Lavender + 1 oz Camellia Oil

Safety

Possible sensitizer- avoid prolonged daily application

Ginger *zingiber officinale*

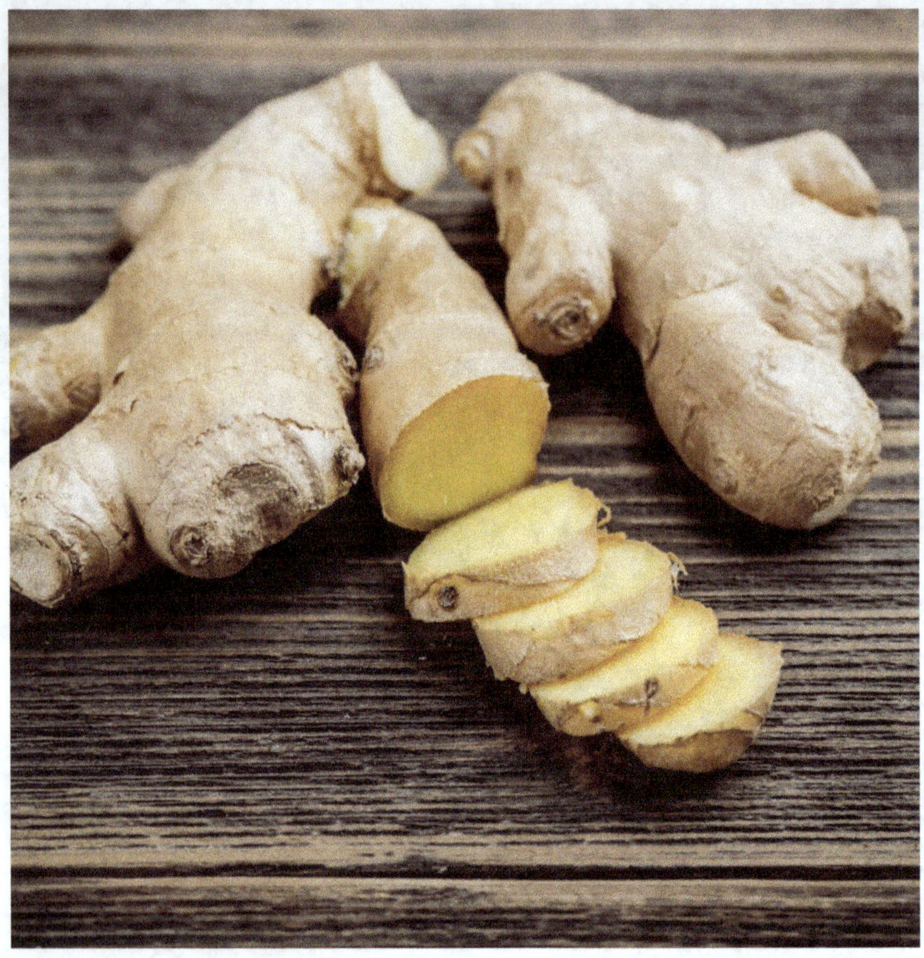

Since ancient times, ginger has been greatly valued for its medicinal properties. With a warm, rich, woodsy, and spicy aroma–it helps to soothe an upset stomach, improve circulation, and alleviate muscle pain.

Background

It is native to the tropics and grows to about 3–4 feet high. The root is used extensively in Asian cuisine and Traditional Chinese Medicine for the treatment of coughs, fevers and nausea. The process of extracting the essential oil begins with macerating the root. Then it is distilled over high heat–extracting the essential oil.

Main Constituents: Sesquiterpenes

Country of origin: Sri Lanka, China, India, Indonesia

Extraction Method: Steam distillation

Part of Plant used: Rhizome

Therapeutics

Add warmth to your massage and revitalize energy and circulation.

Physical:

- Improves Circulation
- Digestive Tonic
- Warming- Cold, damp conditions and cold hands and feet
- Expectorant- congestion
- Analgesic- muscular and joint pain
- Menstrual Pain
- Nausea-motion sickness
- Neuralgia

Emotional:

- Promotes a meditative state of peace and calm
- Sedative
- Antidepressant- sense of worthlessness, self-destruction
- Nervine
- Carminative- anxiety, tension, fear
- Stills the mind-agitation, inability to focus

Blends well with

Ylang Ylang, lemongrass, all citrus oils such as orange, lemon, Frankincense, Lavender, other spice oils such as clove, black pepper and lemongrass.

Bodyworker Applications

Warming Massage Oil: Soothes sore muscles and joints and aids with circulation. 1 oz carrier oil + 5 drops Ginger + 3 drops Frankincense + 2 drops Lavender + 2 drops Sweet Orange

Jet Lag- Aromatherapy Inhaler: 8 drops Grapefruit + 7 drops Ginger

Safety

May cause skin sensitivities, use in high dilution. Avoid with patients showing excess heat signs.

Grapefruit *citrus paradisi*

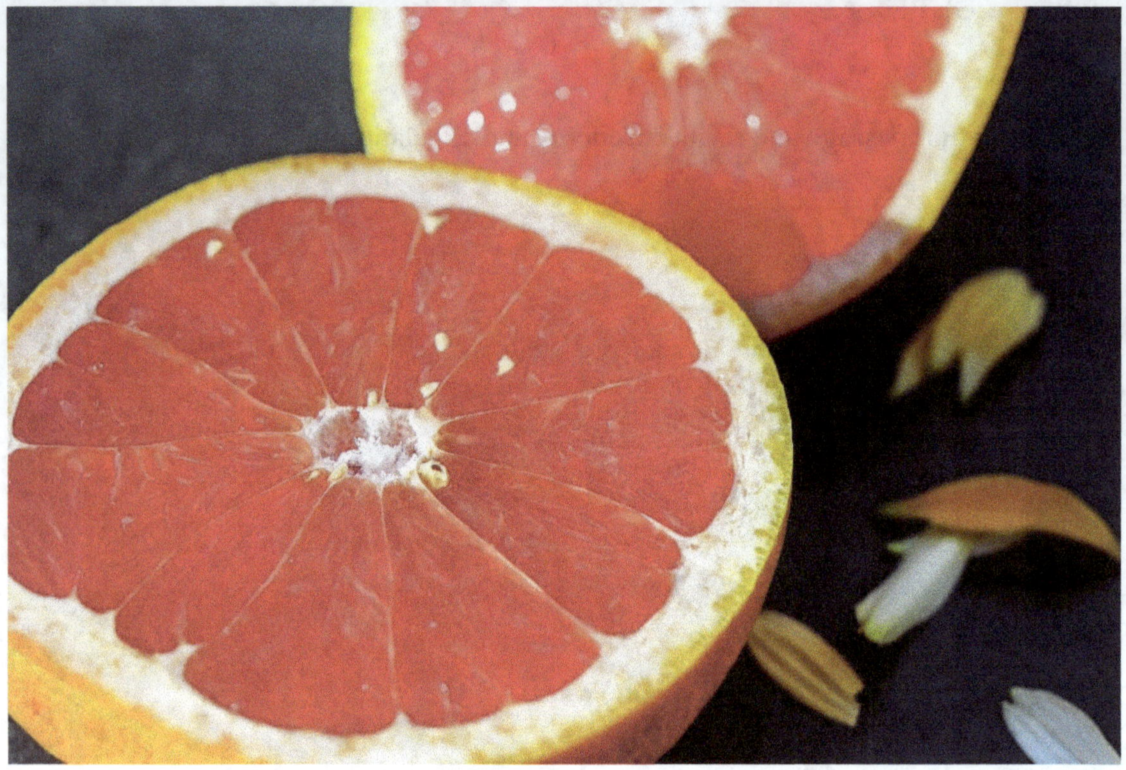

Zesty, bright, sharp, and sweet– grapefruit brightens and revives the spirit. Widely used in skincare and to support lymphatic cleansing.

The smell of grapefruit brings me back to the happy years I worked at a Physiotherapy Wellness Center in Florida. When Citrus was in season, clients would bring bags of grapefruit amongst other citrus fruits. We happily accepted and the smell of grapefruit spread throughout the office. The whole office smelled of Citrus! Our families benefited too as there was so much to go around. They were so delicious!

Background

The grapefruit tree is native to Asia and can grow 16-20 ft tall. It produces a semi bitter-sweet fruit that grows in clusters resembling grapes, which is where it got its name. In 1930, Florida became the first commercial supplier of the essential oil. The US today is still the largest producer in the world. Grapefruits are the result of the cross between two fruits: the sweet orange (Citrus sinensis), itself an ancient hybrid of Asian origin; the other was the Indonesian pomelo (C. maxima).

Grapefruit is an oil of optimism, inviting in a new "zest for life". Emotionally, grapefruit promotes "lightness" and positivity to lift a heavy spirit. It is brightening to the mood and euphoric. It is utilized by Aromatherapist as a "releasing" oil. To help release repressed emotions that can be harmful to your health. It has also been used by aromatherapist for aiding with mood swings, and also helping to balance the appetite. When emotions are dragging, use grapefruit to brighten your day and direct your focus towards the positive, while enhancing confidence and self esteem. Grapefruit Blends beautifully with most oils and will add light, refreshing notes to your aromatherapy blends.

Main Constituents: Up to 95% monoterpenes

Country of origin: Brazil, Argentina, Israeli, South Africa, Spain and the USA

Extraction Method: Cold pressed

Part of Plant used: peel

Therapeutics

Brightens and revives the spirit with optimism to give you a new "Zest for life"

Physical:

- Cleansing to lymphatic system
- Congestion
- Lipolytic- Highest in (+)-Limonene, helps break down fat deposits
- Aids metabolism
- Analgesic
- Antibacterial
- Antioxidant
- Anti-inflammatory
- Skin smoothing, brightening clearing and toning
- Diuretic

Emotional:

- Emotional Balance- repressed emotions
- Uplifting and stimulating
- Restores an overworked or tired nervous system
- Reduces appetite
- Depression- overindulgence or emotional eating
- Releases stress
- Promotes a "lightness of spirit"

Blends well with

Other citrus oils, Lavender, Basil, Rosemary, Peppermint, Geranium, Ylang Ylang, Juniper, Cedarwood.

Bodyworker Applications

Detox Salt Scrub: 5 drops Juniper + 5 drops Grapefruit + 5 drops Orange + 4 oz Sea Salt + 2 oz Fractionated Coconut Oil

Blissful Paradise- Massage Oil: 1 oz Carrier + 3 drops Grapefruit + 3 drops Lime + 2 drops Bergamot 4 drops Ylang Ylang

Safety

Phototoxic. After massaging into the skin, do not expose to strong sun or sunbed for at least 12 hours after application.

Ho Wood *Cinnamomum camphora ct. linalool*

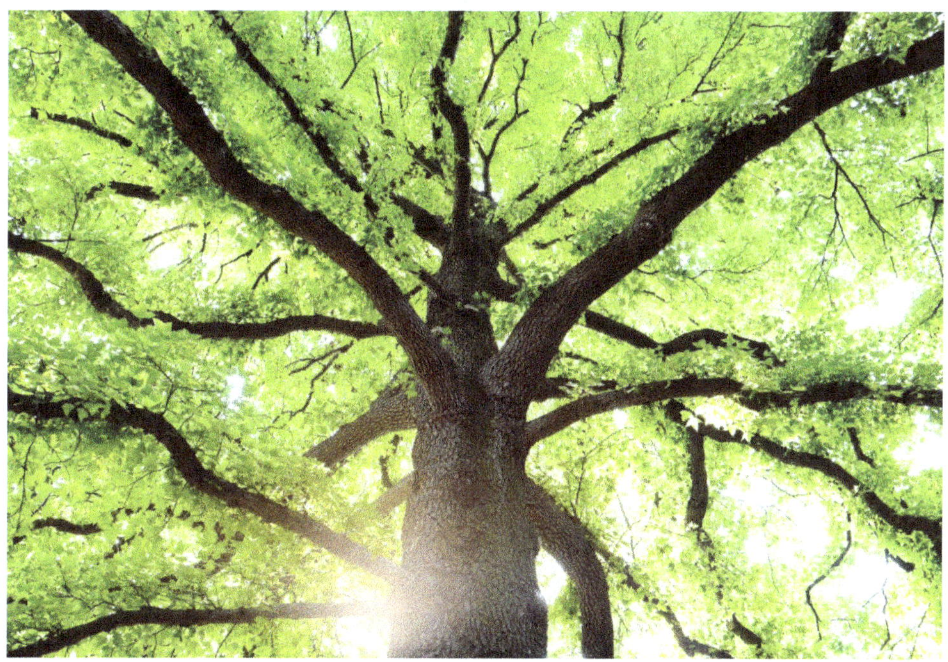

Want to enhance your healing space with a peaceful and relaxing touch? Get to know Ho Wood; your new best friend that promotes a sense of calm to the mind without causing drowsiness. Ho Woods's gift lies in its immense levels of Linalool (one of the highest sources of naturally occurring linalool found in any essential oil), which makes it deeply calming. It is often referred to as the peaceful oil. Its beautiful fragrance and properties are similar and often compared to Rosewood Oil, which is an endangered species and should be avoided. Its aroma is sweet, Woodsy, and rose-like with a hint of camphor.

Background

Did you know that Ho Wood, Ravintsara, and Camphor oils all come from the same tree? Cinnamomum camphora is a large evergreen tree native to the forests of China, Japan, Taiwan and Vietnam. A member of the Lauraceae family, camphor trees are tall evergreens with a spreading canopy made of glossy, bright green aromatic leaves that smell of camphor when crushed. There are six different chemical variants or chemotypes: camphor, linalool, 1,8-cineole, borneol, nerolidol, and safrole. The chemotypes are dependent on the geographical origin of the tree and part of the tree used e.g. leaf or wood/bark.

The essential oil of ho wood ct. linalool, also called "Ho-sho", is steam distilled from the harvested bark, twigs, and wood of the ho wood tree growing in its native habitat.

Note: Ho Wood essential oil is not the same as Ravintsara Essential Oil (ho leaf). Both ho wood and ho leaf come from the same tree, Cinnamomum camphora but they derive from different parts of the plant which makes them different essential oils. Ho Leaf Oil, aka Ravintsara Essential Oil, is distilled from the leaves of the Ho Tree. Ho Wood comes from the bark and wood.

Main Constituents: Linalool: > 98%

Country of origin: China

Extraction Method: Steam distillation

Part of Plant used: bark, twigs, and wood

Therapeutics

Soothing and calming for the mind and body. This restorative tonic promotes mental and emotional balance and is beneficial for reducing inflammation, pain relief, antidepressant, boosting immunity, and promoting skin health.

Physical:

- Analgesic
- Anti-inflammatory
- Antimicrobial
- Antifungal (candida)
- Antioxidant
- Antispasmodic
- Soothes irritated skin (eczema and psoriasis)
- Cooling
- Decongestant

Emotional:

- Antianxiety
- Sedative
- Nervous Tension
- Meditative
- Antidepressant
- Stress-related conditions
- Promotes restful sleep
- Lifts the spirits

Blends well with

Bergamot, Bergamot mint, Lavender, Geranium, clary Sage, and Cedarwood.

Bodyworker Applications

Gentle Massage oil - relieve tension and lift the spirits.

4 drops Ho wood + 4 drops Lavender + 2 drops Mandarin + 1oz carrier oil

Overwhelm Inhaler blend

3 drops Ho Wood + 5 drops Bergamot + 4 drops Clary Sage + 3 drops Mandarin + Aromatherapy Inhaler

Calm and Meditate Synergy - Use the following oils with appropriate dilution in a diffuser, inhaler, massage oil, or bath.

Ho wood + Lavender + Frankincense

Safety

Non-toxic, non-sensitizing, non-irritant. Be sure to purchase Ho Wood from a supplier that has been rectified to remove carcinogenic safrole.

Juniper *juniperus communis*

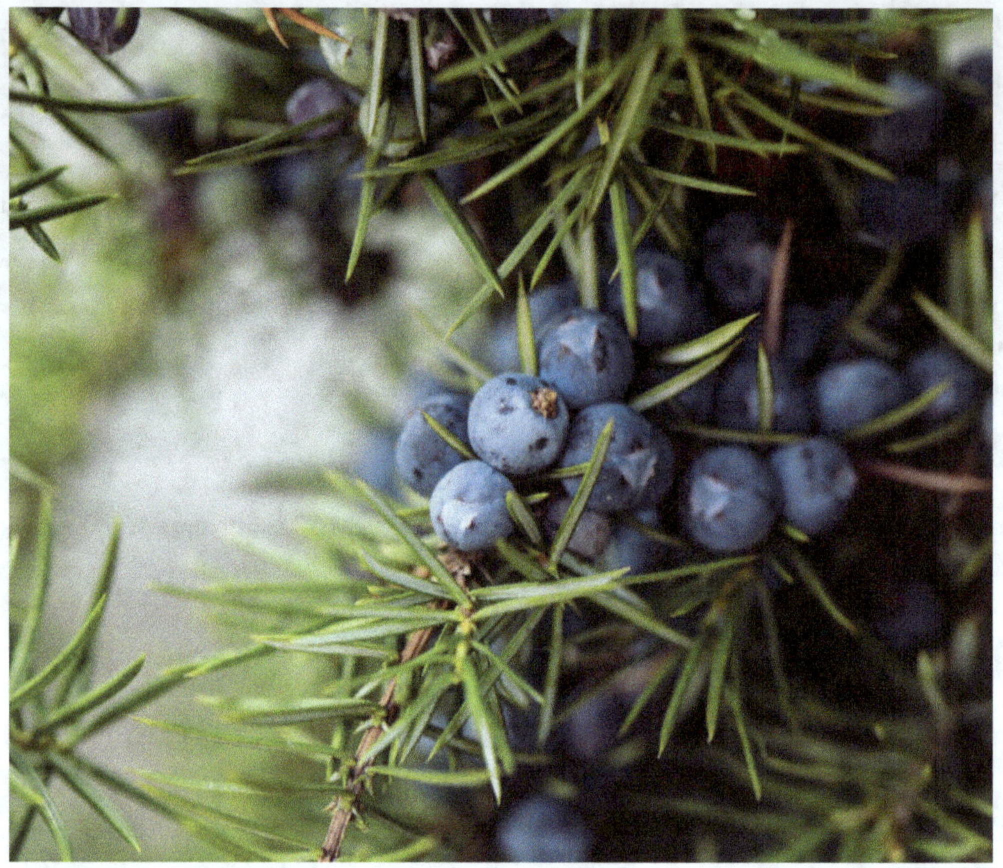

Grounding, calming, and excellent for air purification! The medicine lies in its berries—and just like it purifies the air; it helps to detoxify our organ systems too, especially the kidneys.

Juniper has a fresh, peppery, and woodsy aroma that becomes softer and sweeter as it evaporates.

Background

The common Juniper is a coniferous evergreen shrub or tree that can grow from 6-25 feet.

Juniper was burned in ancient Greek as an air purifier and used by the ancient Egyptians in the mummification process. All of the aerial parts can be used; however, the berries are considered the most therapeutic.

In traditional medicine, Juniper berries were often used to treat urinary tract infections, kidney stones, and to promote detoxification by eliminating excess fluids and toxins from the body.

Central Europeans consume Juniper berries as a preserve to boost their immune system and use them as a key ingredient in flavoring gin. Native Americans have used Juniper to treat muscle aches, arthritis, cold and flus.

Main Constituents: Monoterpenes

Principal Places of Production: Italy, France, Spain, Hungary, India, Croatia, USA

Part of Plant used: Ripe berries

Extraction method: Steam Distillation

Therapeutics

Support detoxification and cleansing of the body and mind.

Physical:

- Warming
- Superior Detoxifier
- Diuretic
- Antirheumatic
- Circulatory Tonic- cold limbs
- Congested skin
- Warming and Stimulating- Yang
-
- Anti-inflammatory
- Antispasmodic

Emotional:

- Mentally refreshing-fatigue, concentration
- Psychological stagnation
- Fluctuating energy levels
- Emotionally frozen
- Coldness
- Lack of motivation
- Feeling "blocked"
- Emotional Fortitude- worry, overwhelm

Blends well with

Rosemary, Lavender, citrus oils such as Bergamot, Lime and Grapefruit, Eucalyptus, Geranium, Ginger, Black Pepper.

Bodyworker Applications

Relieve my Aches Bath- Daytime Bath: 2 drops Juniper + 2 drops Lavender + 2 drops Cypress + 2 drops Rosemary + 1 tsp carrier oil + 1 tbsp Castile soap

Muscle Strain Oil: 5 drops Juniper + 5 drops Rosemary + 2 drops Black Pepper + 4 drops Clary Sage + 4 drops Chamomile + 2 oz Carrier Oil

Lymph Mover massage Oil: 5 drops Juniper + 5 drops Grapefruit + 5 drops Geranium + 1 oz. carrier oil or unscented lotion

Safety

Avoid use when kidney disease is present, acute bladder infections, or during pregnancy. Non- to mildly sensitizing. Do not take Juniper berry essential oil internally.

Lavender *lavandula angustifolia*

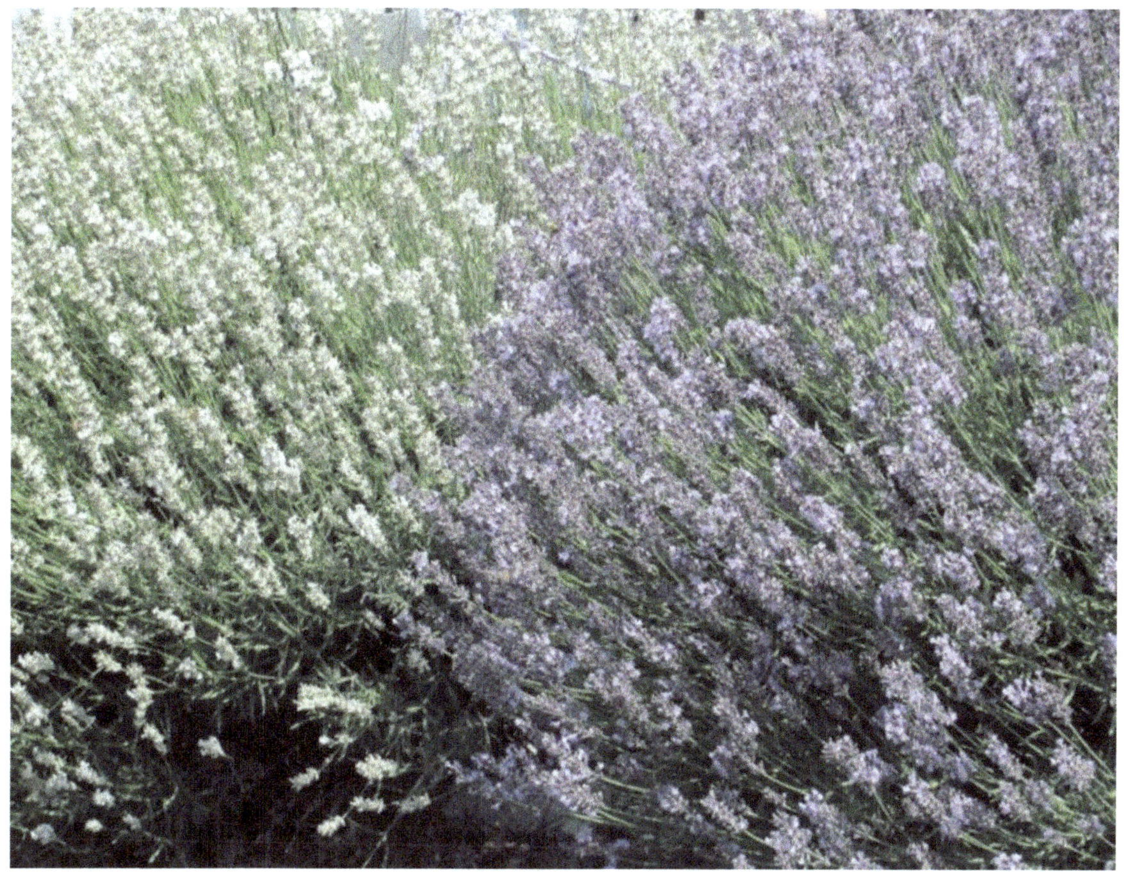

"Look to the nervous system as the key to maximum health."- Galen

She's well loved, with good reason. Lavender is a powerful antimicrobial, anxiolytic, anti-inflammatory, antinociceptive, and antioxidant. Lavender is sometimes referred to as a "first aid kit in a bottle" because of its versatility.

One of the most popular essential oils–lavender is gentle, calming, helps with anxiety, and her aroma is fresh, floral, herbaceous, and sweet.

Background

The Latin name for lavender is "lavare" which means to wash. Owing to its pleasant and clean scent, it was utilized by the Romans for bathing and cleansing their homes.

Lavender is one of the most popular essential oils used for calming the nerves. It is gentle and has many uses. Lavandula angustifolia essential oils will vary a slight bit in terms of constituent percentages, but all of them can be used interchangeably.

Main Constituents: Esters, linalool and linalyl acetate

Principal Places of Production: France, England, Bulgaria, USA

Part of Plant used: Flowering tops

Extraction method: Steam distillation

Therapeutics

There is practically no health condition for which lavender would not provide some kind of relief for. Like a warm, soft blanket–lavender invokes feelings of security.

Physical:

- Muscle Spasms
- Bug bites
- Anti-inflammatory
- Nervine
- Diuretic
- Nervous digestive upsets
- Muscular Aches
- Bursitis
- Burns
- Skincare-promotes cell growth, balance sebum production
- Wound healing
- Inflamed skin conditions
- Neuralgia
- Insect repellant

Emotional:

- Extreme emotional changes- helps promote mental peace and balance
- Anxiety and nervous tension
- Can aid with restful sleep
- TCM- supports Qi-energy of the heart
- Restlessness
- Calms, relaxes, and restores the nervous system

- Fear of touch
- Trauma
- Reduces agitation and anger

Blends well with

Most oils, especially to harmonize a blend.

Bodyworker Applications

Neck Tension Oil: 10 drops Lavender + 4 drops Rosemary + 6 drops Peppermint + 1 oz carrier oil

Stress Reducer Massage Oil: 4 drops Lavender + 4 drops Orange + 3 drops Cedarwood + 2 drops Lime + 1 oz carrier oil

Safety

Non-irritant, non-phototoxic, non-toxic.

Lemongrass *cymbopogon citratus*

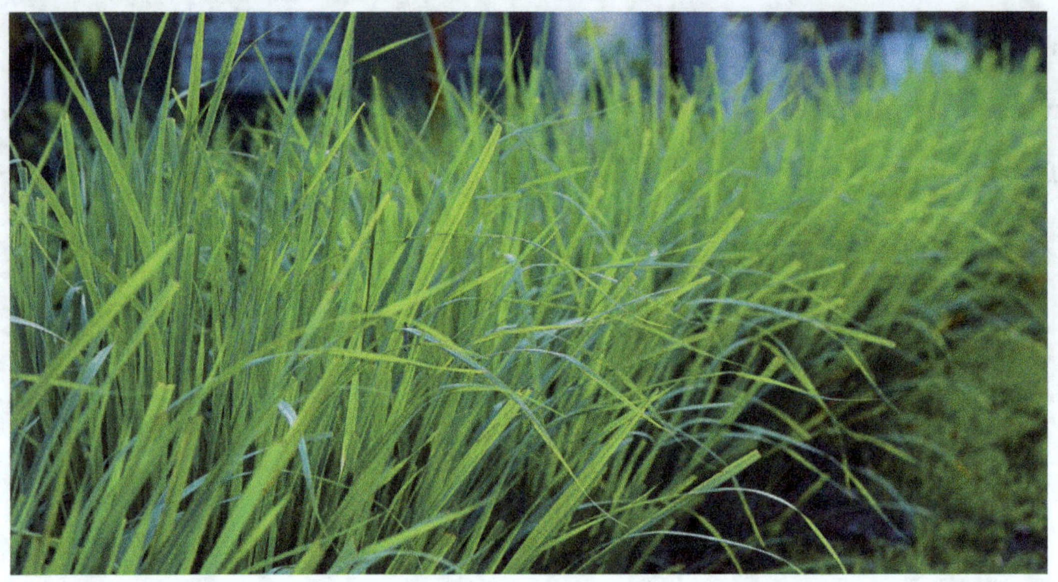

Besides having the most delightful, earthy, lemon-y aroma, lemongrass is a phenomenal aid for digestive issues and high blood pressure/cholesterol. It also is incredibly stimulating and energizing when your nervous system needs a pick me up.

Background

The word for Lemongrass in Sanskrit is "Bhu-trna" which means "earth grass". West Indian lemongrass grows up to 5 ft tall.

Its aromatic "blades" can cut you if you are not careful. It is a common ingredient in Thai cuisine and serves as a flavoring agent across Asian nations. It finds extensive application in TCM and Ayurvedic medicine. Often found in citrus-scented perfumes and soaps, it also works as an insect repellent.

Main Constituents: Rich in the aldehydes (up to 80%) and monoterpenes

Principal Places of Production: India, Madagascar, Brazil, Malaysia and Vietnam

Part of Plant used: Grass

Extraction method: Steam Distillation

Therapeutics

"Lemongrass enables to mind to shift towards fascination about what is possible, encouraging you to embark on a glorious voyage of discovery." -The Blossoming Heart by Robbi Zeck, ND

Physical:

- Antifungal
- Digestive Soother
- Nerve pain
- Restores the nervous system
- Muscular pain, strains, bruises
- Tired, sore, fatigued muscles
- Strengthens weak connective tissue
- Poor, sluggish circulation
- Varicose veins
- Headaches
- Abdominal pain

Emotional:

- Emotional restrictions
- Nervous restorative
- Fatigue
- Strengthening during transitional period
- Grieving process
- Release work
- Elevates the mood
- Promotes Mental Clarity

Blends well with

Eucalyptus, Bergamot, Fennel, Geranium, Ginger, Lavender, Lemon, Mandarin, Peppermint, Rosemary, Tea tree

Bodyworker Applications

Over Exercised Muscles: 5 drops Lemongrass + 4 drops Ginger + 6 drops Lavender + 5 drops Rosemary + 4 drops Peppermint + 2 oz carrier oil or Arnica infused oil.

Emotional Equilibrium Diffuser Blend: Lemongrass + Lavender + Atlas Cedarwood

Antibacterial Cleansing Spray: Use to disinfect countertops and other surfaces. Contains alcohol- keep away from open flames.

Add essential oils first to a 4 oz glass, PET plastic or aluminum bottle with atomizer. Then add 190 (95%) proof Alcohol. Mix. Then add water, or your favorite hydrosol.

Fill the bottle with a minimum of 20-30% 150 Proof Alcohol (such as ever clear), then the remaining with water.

20 drops Lemongrass + 20 drops Orange + 20 drops Eucalyptus + 20 drops Tea Tree

Safety

Avoid undiluted application. Do not use in the bath, or on sensitive, damaged or allergy prone skin.

Lime *citrus aurantifolia*

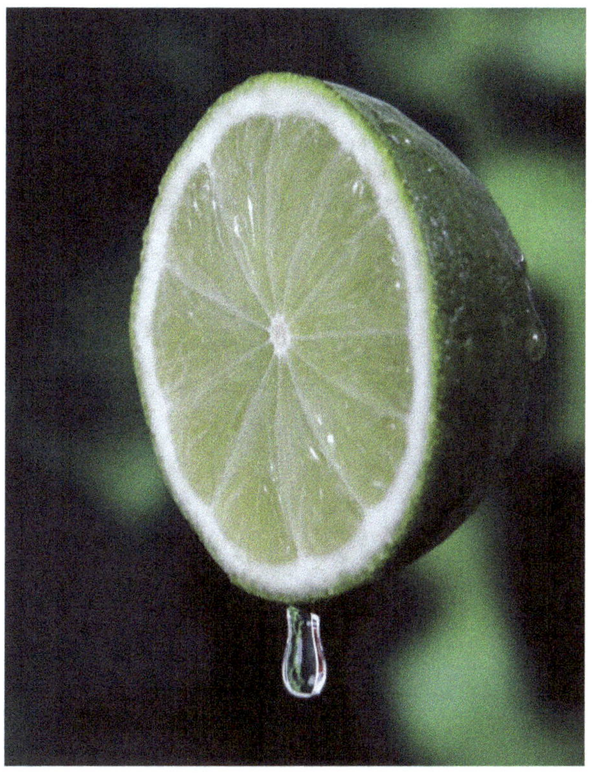

"The lime trees were in bloom. But in the early morning only a faint fragrance drifted through the garden, an airy message, an aromatic echo of the dreams during the short summer night."
- Isak Dinesen

Lime is your seemingly always bright and happy best friend. Its tantalizing aroma is fresh, bright, awakens the senses, and lifts the spirit. Commonly used as a natural cleaning agent, and as an astringent and toner for the skin.

Background

The lime tree, originally from Asia, made its way to Europe thanks to the Moors. Limes contain vitamin C (ascorbic acid) and the British navy formerly used them to prevent scurvy, which is why they were nicknamed "limey" or "lime juicers".

Christopher Columbus took citrus seeds, probably including limes, to the West Indies on his second voyage in 1493, and the trees soon became widely distributed in the West Indies, Mexico, and Florida. It has a higher acid and sugar content than Lemons.

Limes find their use in the beverage industry, as well as in perfumes, deodorants, and aftershaves.

Main Constituents: Limonene

Principal Places of Production: Asia, Mexico, South Africa, USA, Italy

Part of Plant used: Peel

Extraction method: Cold Press, steam distillation

Therapeutics

Enhance mental clarity and cleanse your body and mind with its bright, zesty scent!

Physical:

- Astringent and toning- oily skin
- Cooling
- Digestive stimulant
- Infections, fever, colds
- Detoxifying

Emotional:

- Elevates the mood- promotes feelings of positivity, calm and harmony.
- Anxiety, depression
- Apathy- awakens the spirit
- Refreshes and uplifts a tired mind
- Energizing

Blends well with

Eucalyptus, Bergamot, Geranium, Lavender, Grapefruit, Orange, Peppermint, Rosemary, Tea tree, Basil, Rosemary, Cedarwood, and Clary sage

Bodyworker Applications

Zestful Zen Synergy: Soothe the nerves and reduce stress and tension. Diffuse, or use as a massage oil diluted with a carrier. Lime + Grapefruit + Lavender.

Lime Oasis - **An anxiety reducing massage oil:** 3 drops Lime + 2 drops Orange + 3 drops Vetiver + 3 drops Bergamot + 1 oz. carrier oil. Can be added to a roller bottle for support on the go.

Safety

Expressed lime is phototoxic. Do not use before going into the sun or UV light. Steam distilled lime is ok.

Mandarin *Citrus reticulata*

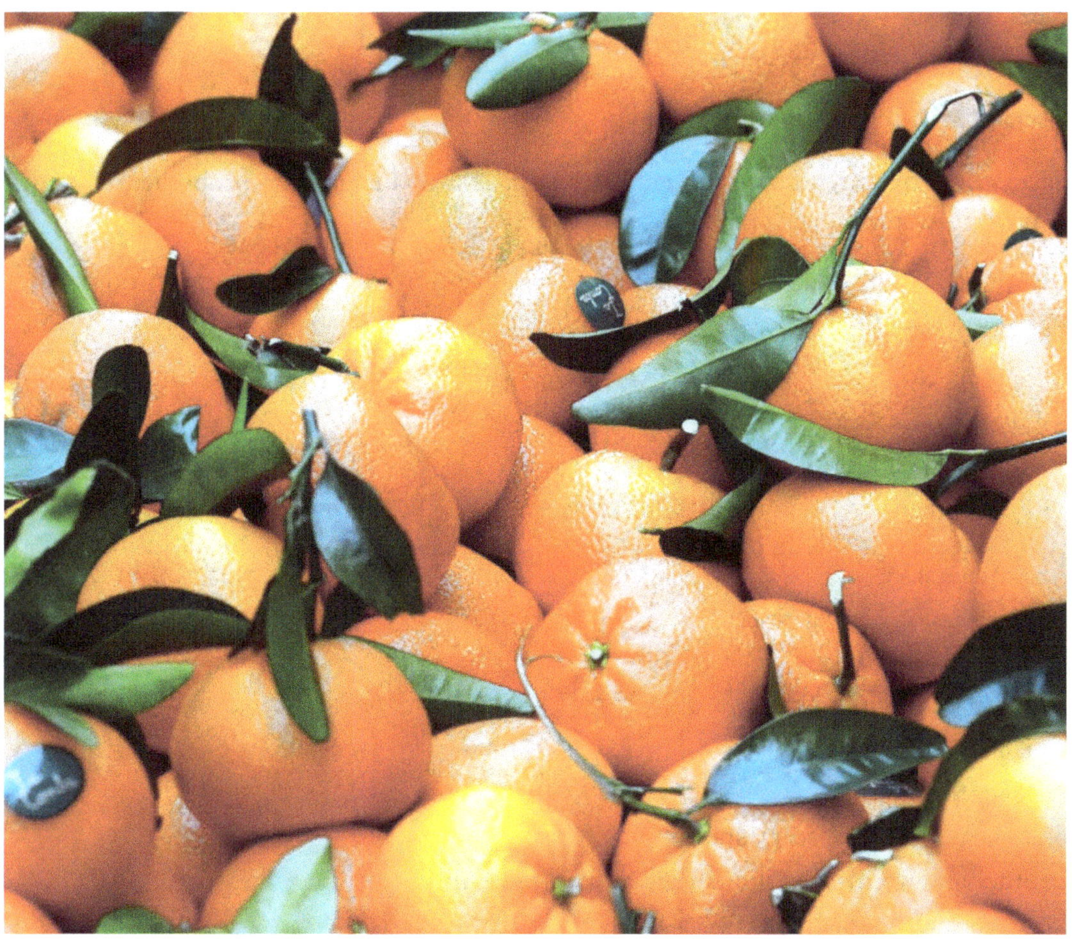

"He who laughs at himself never runs out of things to laugh at." - Epictetus

The vibrant zing of Mandarin essential oil is a true gem for anyone chasing down peace in both their physical and mental realms. Its sunny fragrance is calming and positive, helping to disarm a shielding nervous system. There's something sweet and innocent about these little citrus fruits.

Background

The history of mandarin fruit dates back thousands of years to ancient China, where it is believed to have originated. People in China have cultivated mandarins for over 3,000 years and highly valued them as fruits in the imperial courts. They were a popular choice for gifts and were commonly used in traditional Chinese medicine for their various health benefits.

Main Constituents: Limonene: 80% +

Country of origin: China

Extraction Method: Cold press

Part of Plant used: Rind

Therapeutics

Mandarin essential oil is renowned for its soothing and mood-enhancing properties, which make it a favored option in aromatherapy practices.

It is said to help "bring out the inner child", and can help reduce stress, anxiety, promotes relaxation, and brings comfort to the mind, body and heart (Shen).

Physical:

- Antiseptic
- Antimicrobial
- Analgesic
- Antibacterial
- Improves blood circulation
- Warming
- Anti-inflammatory
- Antispasmodic
- Astrigent
- Skin- acne, oily skin, scars, spots
- Soothes and warms sore joints-rheumatism and arthritis.
- Digestive aid
- Decongest lymphatics
- Detoxifier
- Hepatic
- Immune system tonic

Emotional:

- Anti-anxiety
- Sedative - Insomnia
- Stress- nervous tension

- Meditative
- Antidepressant
- Stress-related conditions
- Emotional trauma
- Listless
- Lifts the spirits

Blends well with

Other citrus oils, Ginger, Lavender, Clary Sage, Geranium, Cedarwood, Bergamot Mint, Yarrow, and Ylang Ylang.

Bodyworker Applications

Post Partum Massage oil -For postpartum fatigue and adjusting to motherhood.

3 drops Lavender + 2 drops Rosemary + 3 drops Mandarin + 2 drops Geranium + 1 oz carrier oil

Slumber Diffuser blend

Clary Sage + Mandarin + Lavender

Couples Massage OIl

10 drops Mandarin + 3 drops of Ylang Ylang + 4 drops of Ho Wood + 1 oz of Almond Oil

Alluring Body Salt Scrub

25 drops Mandarin + 5 drops Vetiver + 10 drops Rose Geranium + 8 oz Pink Himalayan Salt + 4-8oz Fractionated Coconut Oil (adjust depending how oily or dry you want it)

Safety

If the oil is old and oxidized it may cause skin irritation. Use at a 1% dilution for sensitive skin.

Sweet Orange *citrus sinensis*

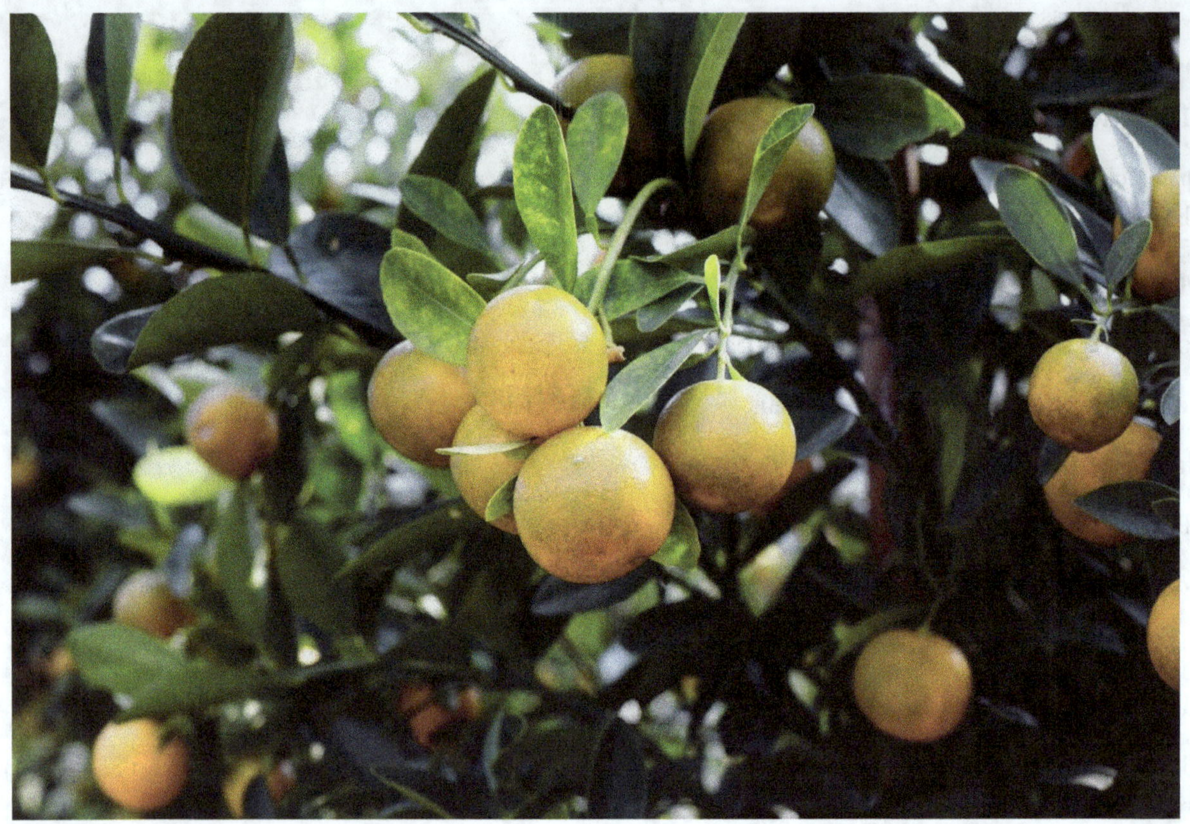

"Misery might love company, but so does joy. And joy throws much better parties."–Billy Ivey

Sweet orange essential oil will give your skin a glow while simultaneously infusing your spirit with vitality. A staple aromatherapy oil for creating a bright, uplifting and invigorating ambiance.

Background

The sweet orange tree can grow between 24 to 49 feet. It has many soft green leaves and its flowers are white and fragrant. It produces a delicious orange sphere shaped fruit that is used as a flavoring in confections and a fragrance note in perfumes, soaps and other toiletries.

Sweet Orange had its origin in India and Portuguese sailors brought it back to Europe, from where they carried it to South America.

Main Constituents: Rich in monoterpenes

Principal Places of Production: Brazil, United States, Italy, Spain, Argentina.

Part of Plant used: Peel

Extraction method: Cold Pressed

Therapeutics

Its warm, sunny aroma enlivens the mood, inspires the mind, reduces stress, and promotes relaxation, making it beneficial for formulations focused on mental well-being. When diluted in a carrier, it can be used topically to enhance skin health, as it possesses antibacterial properties, aids in reducing inflammation, and refreshes our body systems.

Physical:

- Promotes detoxification
- Skin toning and cleansing
- Stimulates the Lymphatic System
- Soothing to the nerves
- Warming
- Neutralizes microbes
- Promotes sleep
- Carminative

Emotional:

- Enlivens
- Mood enhancer and relaxant
- Balances the mind and body
- Uplifting
- Worry-reducing
- Cheerful
- Relieves anxiety

Blends well with

Geranium, Clary Sage, Vetiver, Palma Rosa, Cedarwood, Geranium, Ylang Ylang, Lavender, other citrus oils such as Lime, Grapefruit, Bergamot, and spice oils such as Cinnamon, Clove and Ginger.

Bodyworker Applications

Freshen Citrus - Tea Tree Cleaning Spray:

Ratio for Castile soap to water: ¼ c. (60 mL) soap in a quart (1 L) of water in a spray bottle.

Add essential oils to the bottle first, then castile soap, then water. 40 drops Sweet Orange + 40 drops Lime + 20 drops Tea Tree

Sleep Deprived Blend: Blend the following in an essential oil atomizer bottle. Add 1-2 drops to a tissue and place it near your pillow to aid falling asleep. 10 drops Lavender + 5 drops Clary Sage + 5 drops Sweet Orange

Emotional Balance (for sadness, grief): 10 drops Orange + 9 drops Cypress Oil + 8 drops Frankincense + 3 drops Geranium + 1 oz Carrier Oil

Safety

Non-irritant, non-sensitizing. Use less than 7-10 drops citrus oils, singly or combined in the bath to avoid potential skin irritation.

Palmarosa *Cymbopogon martinii*

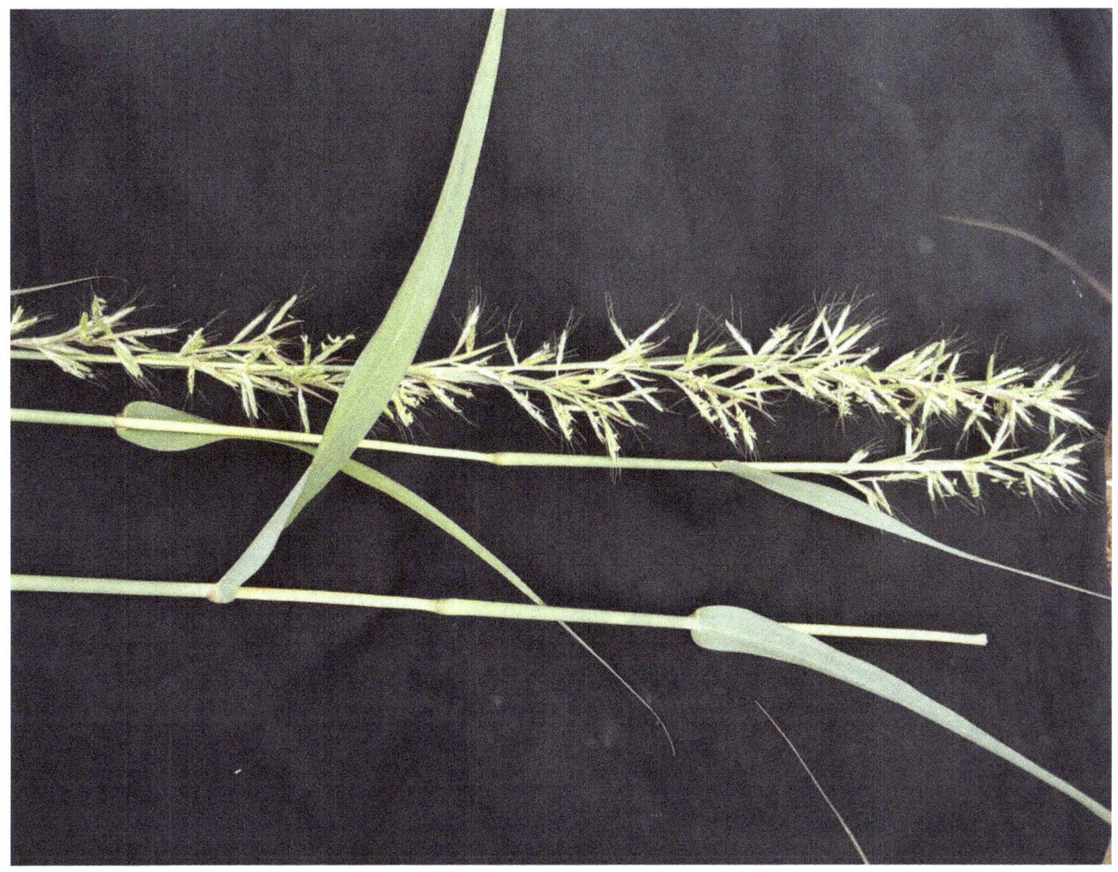

"It is compassion, then, that is the best protection; it is also, as the great masters of the past have always known, the source of all healing." - Sogyal Rinpoche

Palmarosa invites you to a tropical paradise. It takes you through a journey of compassion, to heal a wounded spirit and lift daily stresses away. Its this soft, green, and floral essence is often considered similar to Gcare eranium, yet more subtle. However, a little goes a long way with this oil!

Background

Palmarosa, scientifically known as Cymbopogon martinii, is a fragrant grass native to India and other parts of Southeast Asia. It belongs to the same genus as lemongrass and citronella. Historically, palmarosa has been used for various purposes, and its essential oil offers numerous benefits for the mind and body.

Palmarosa has a long history of use in Ayurvedic medicine, the traditional medicine of India- where it was valued for its antiseptic, antibacterial, and antifungal properties.

It is used to treat skin infections, digestive issues, and fever. The dried leaves of palmarosa were also traditionally used as a fragrant addition to potpourris and sachets.

Palmarosa essential oil is sometimes referred to as "Indian geranium oil" due to its similar aroma to geranium oil. The name "palmarosa" is derived from the Latin words "palma," meaning palm tree, and "rosa," meaning rose, referring to the plant's resemblance to both palm and rose. The grass of the palmarosa plant is steam distilled to extract its essential oil, which ranges in color from pale yellow to amber and has a sweet, floral scent reminiscent of rose with citrus undertones.

Main Constituents: geraniol, geranyl acetate, linalool, citronellol, and dipentene.

Country of origin: India

Extraction Method: Steam distillation

Part of Plant used: Grass

Therapeutics

Take in the aroma of Palmarosa to support you during stressful periods and times of anxiety, grief, anger or general nervous tension. Palmarosa essential oil is renowned for its skincare benefits. It is commonly used in skincare products due to its ability to balance sebum production, making it suitable for both oily and dry skin types. It also has hydrating and rejuvenating properties that can help improve the appearance of the skin and reduce the signs of aging.

Physical:

- Sinusitis
- Excess Mucus
- Cystitis
- Antimicrobial
- Urinary Tract Infection
- Gastrointestinal Disorders
- Scars
- Wounds
- Acne
- Boils
- Fungal Infection

- Muscular Aches -Over-excercised Muscles
- Insect Bites And Stings
- Deodorizing

Emotional:

- General FatigueAntianxiety
- Stress
- Anxiety- nervous tension
- Irritability
- Restlessness
- Calming

Blends well with

Lavender, Geranium, clary Sage, Bergamot, Orange, Mandarin, Ylang Ylang, Vetiver, and Cedarwood.

Bodyworker Applications:

Tranquility Fusion Massage oil - Relieve tension, and lift the spirits.

9 drops of Bergamot Mint + 4 drops Vetiver Oil + 3 drops Lavender Oil

2 drops of Mandarin + 1 oz Castor oil (or 50% castor oil & 50% carrier of choice)

Mood Calm - Inhaler blend

4 drops Palmarosa + 5 drops Bergamot + 5 drops Lavender + 3 drops Sweet Orange + Aromatherapy Inhaler

Be Still Massage Butter

15 drops Palmarosa + 10 Ho Wood + 10 drops Frankincense + 6 drops Vetiver + 4oz Whipped Massage Butter

Safety

Non-toxic, non-irritating. According to Essential Oil Safety by Tisserand and Young (second edition), in spite of European legislation listing geraniol as an allergen, the risk of geraniol allergy is very low. Tisserand recommends maximum topical use of 6.5%.

Peppermint *mentha piperita*

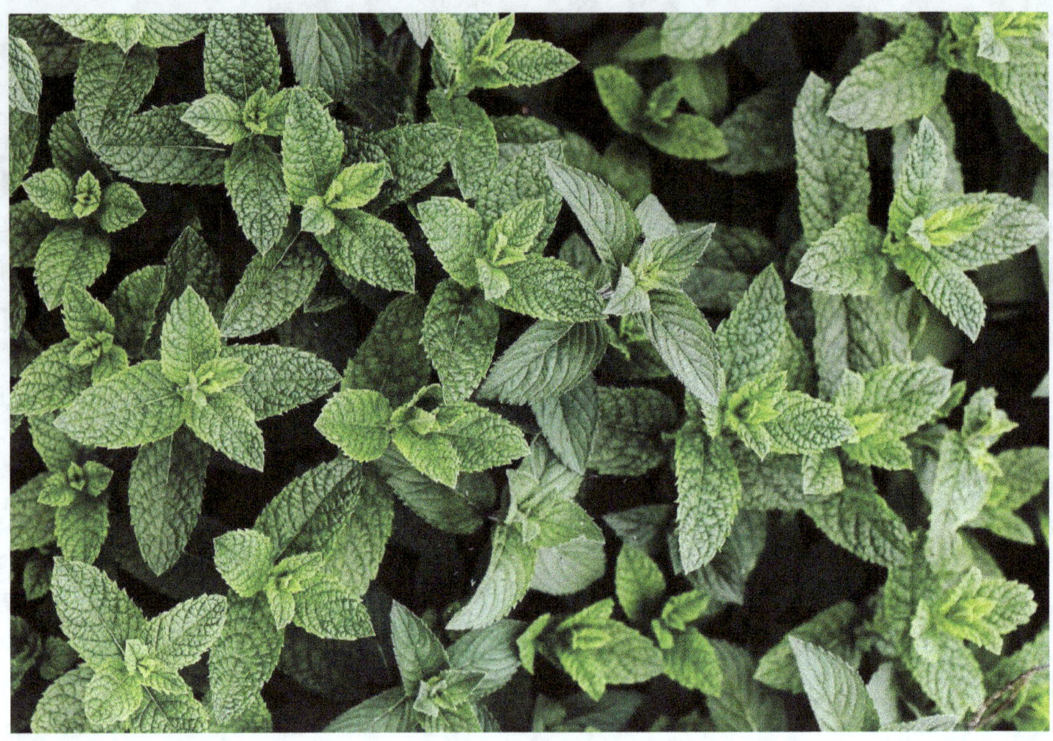

Beneficial for the belly, and energizing for the thoughts. Peppermint essential oil helps to soothe fatigued muscles and is a great oil to work in with athletes.

Background

Mentha piperita is a hybrid of watermint (M. aquatica) and spearmint (M. spicata). The herb can grow up to 3 ft in height and has dark green leaves and tall spikes of purplish flowers. Native to southern Europe, Peppermint is now cultivated in more temperate climates all over the world and was first brought to the USA in the early 19th century.

The US is now the largest producer of peppermint. Mentha piperita has been found in Egyptian tombs dating back to 1000 BC, and there is evidence that peppermint has a long history in Europe, China, and Japan. The Romans loved mint. They wove it into garlands and wore it at feats and used in sauces. Mints appear in early medieval plant lists and they were brought to Britain during the Roman Times.

Main Constituents: Menthol, methone

Principal Places of Production: USA, India, France, England Part of Plant used: Leaves

Extraction method: Steam distillation

Therapeutics

Dramatically opens the breath, awakens the mind and refreshes a tired body.

Physical:

- Muscle stiffness/aches
- Cramping
- Hot Flashes
- Sunburns (use w/Lavender)
- Headaches
- Respiratory support- sinus, congestion
- Stomach upsets- gas, cramps, travel sickness

Emotional:

- Energizes and invigorates
- Expansive essential oil- mind
- Mental Fatigue
- Sluggishness
- Overwork
- Lethargy
- Mental Strain
- Exercise
- Aids in Concentration (use with Rosemary)

Blends well with

Rosemary, Tea Tree, Lavender, Lime, Clary Sage, Eucalyptus, Lemongrass, Orange, Plai, Black Pepper.

Bodyworker Applications

Diffuse to increase concentration or for a "sleepy mind"

Invigorating Body Scrub: ½ cup raw sugar, ¼ cup Carrier Oil, 6 drops Peppermint + 3 drops Lemongrass + 4 drops Lime

Migraine Relief: 6 drops Peppermint + 7 drops Frankincense + 4 drops Lavender + 1 oz carrier oil

Safety

Non-toxic and non-irritating, however peppermint may be sensitizing because of its high menthol content, causing irritation to the skin and mucous membranes. Do not use on children younger than 7 years of age. Do not take internally and avoid using undiluted.

Scotch Pine *Pinus sylvestris*

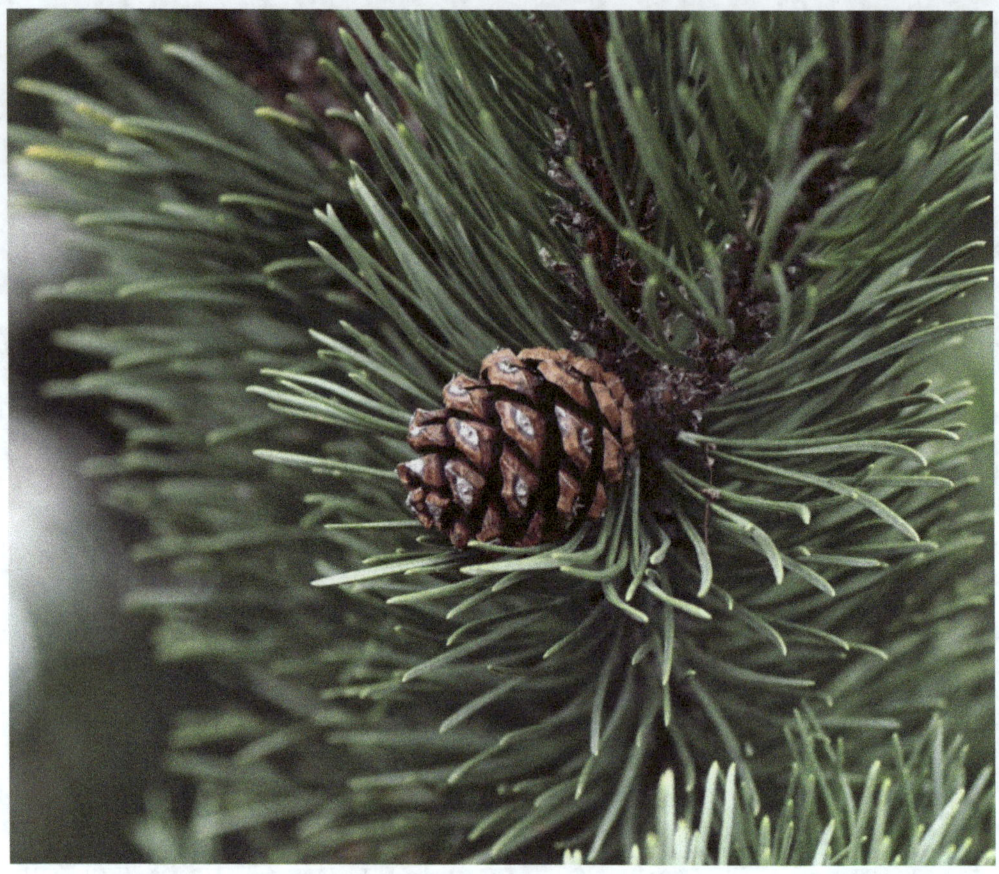

Scotch Pine essential oil offers a personalized retreat to the tranquil depths of the forest, where its restorative properties rejuvenate both mind and body. Take an inspiring walk in the forest with the fresh, earthy, balsamic aroma of pine.

Background

Scotch Pine, scientifically known as Pinus sylvestris, is a species of pine tree native to Europe and Asia. It is one of the most widely distributed pine species in the world and is commonly found across northern and central Europe, Scandinavia, Russia, and parts of Asia. Scotch Pine is known for its resilience and ability to thrive in a variety of environmental conditions, from coastal dunes to mountain slopes.

In traditional European folk medicine, people used Scotch Pine internally as a remedy for respiratory infections, coughs, and colds. Herbal teas made from the young shoots and needles were believed to have therapeutic benefits.

Forest bathing, also known as shinrin-yoku in Japanese, is the practice of immersing oneself in a forest environment to promote physical, mental, and emotional well-being. It involves mindfully spending time in nature, engaging all the senses to connect with the natural world. Engaging in forest bathing reduces stress, lowers blood pressure, boosts the immune system, improves mood, and enhances overall feelings of well-being, according to studies.

Evergreen essential oils, derived from trees such as Pine, Spruce, Fir, and Cedar, capture the essence of the forest and help bring the experience of forest bathing to you, even if you're unable to physically be in a forest.

Main Constituents: Monoterpenes

Country of origin: Scotland, Austria, France, Bulgaria, United States

Extraction Method: Steam distillation

Part of Plant used: Needles

Therapeutics

With its soothing aroma and potent therapeutic qualities, Scotch Pine provides relief for tired muscles and joints while clearing the airways for effortless breathing, fostering a sense of vitality and well-being. Its ability to restore an overworked nervous system is profound.

Physical:

- Analgesic
- Antispasmodic
- Antiinfectious
- Balsamic
- Diuretic
- Decongestant
- Anti-inflammatory
- Antirheumatic
- Antifungal (candida)
- Sinusitis
- Mucolytic

- Tonic
- Muscular fatigue and injury
- Rheumatism
- Circulatory stimulant- warms chilly limbs, cold hands and feet

Emotional:

- Restorative
- Stress relief
- General Debility
- Fatigue
- Mental And Nervous Exhaustion

Blends well with

Bergamot, Copaiba, Chamomile, Cypress, Cedarwood, Lavender, Lemongrass, Juniper, Peppermint, Black Pepper, Nutmeg, Lime, Orange, Rosemary, Eucalyptus, Tea Tree, and Yarrow.

Bodyworker Applications

Heavy Leg Oil - for swelling/edema

5 drops Scotch Pine + 4 drops Grapefruit + 6 drops Cypress + 1 oz carrier oil

Breathe Easy Inhaler

6 drops Pine + 4 drops Peppermint + 5 drops Eucalyptus + Aromatherapy Inhaler

Chest soother- respiratory support

3 drops Scotch Pine + 4 drops Atlas Cedarwood + 4 drops Cypress + 1 oz carrier oil

Restorative Massage Oil- for mental and physical fatigue.

5 drops Scotch Pine + 4 drops Lavender + 4 drops Cypress + 2 drops Black Pepper + 1 oz Carrier oil

Safety

May cause skin irritation on sensitive individuals.. In this case, use in low dilution (5-6 drops per ounce of carrier) when applying to the skin, such as in bath or massage oils.

Plai *Zingiber cassumunar*

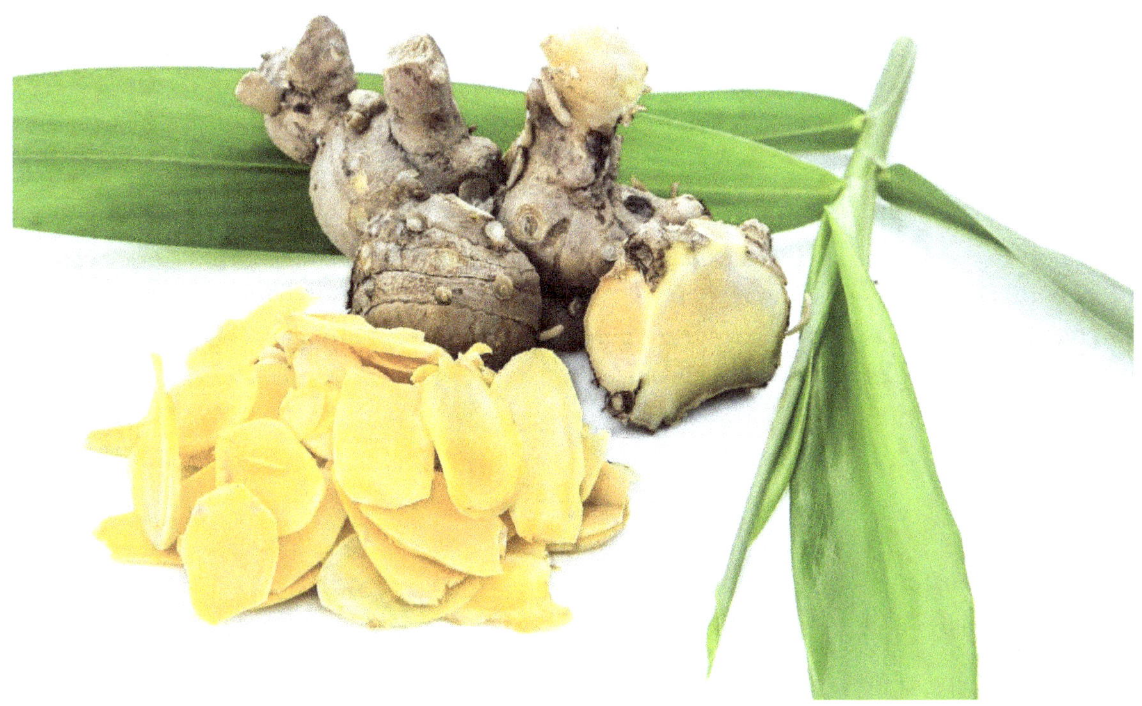

Plai essential oil stands out as its earthy aroma of fresh peppery notes takes you to Thailand, where it is from. It soothes your sore joints and relieves muscular tension from long hikes in the mountains and injuries.

Background

Plai (Zingiber cassumunar), also known as "Cassumunar ginger," is a perennial herbaceous plant native to Southeast Asia, particularly Thailand. It belongs to the ginger family, Zingiberaceae, and is renowned for its medicinal properties.

In traditional Thai medicine, the root of Plai has been used for centuries due to its diverse therapeutic benefits. Practitioners of Traditional Thai Medicine often use the root of Plai topically in various forms, such as poultices, balms (yellow balm), and oils, to alleviate various ailments. It is one of the principal ingredients used in Luk Pra Kob, the Thai Herbal Poultice. This bundle of Thai herbs is steamed and applied to the body, with massage to alleviate sore muscles and joints while sedating the nervous system.

With its legendary healing properties, Plai has been a trusted ally in traditional remedies for treating various ailments such as muscle and joint discomfort, arthritis, rheumatism, sprains, digestive and respiratory issues. It is also used to promote relaxation, making it popular among Thai massage therapists.

Main Constituents: sesquiterpenoids and monoterpenoids

Country of origin: Thailand

Extraction Method: Steam distillation

Part of Plant used: Root

Therapeutics

Unlike the common Ginger, Plai is cooling. When applied topically, Plai root extract exhibits anti-inflammatory, analgesic, and antimicrobial properties. This makes it effective in reducing pain and inflammation associated with musculoskeletal conditions and injuries. It soothes sore, warm, puffy areas, overworked muscles and strain. It is known to have long-lasting analgesic properties that may provide relief for up to 24 hours. An anti-inflammatory, fights septic inflammation, heals bruises and wounds. Use Plai to enhance circulation and stimulate blood flow to affected areas, to aid in the healing process.

Physical:

- Analgesic
- Anti-inflammatory
- Antimicrobial
- Headaches
- Arthritis/rheumatism
- Muscle strain and aches
- Tendonitis
- Increases circulation
- Digestion
- Decongestant
- Neuropathy

Emotional:

- Stress relief
- Clarity
- Focus
- Grounding
- Anxiety

Blends well with

Lemongrass, Ginger, Peppermint, Black Pepper, Lime, Orange, Rosemary, Eucalyptus, Clove.

Bodyworker Applications

Sabai Massage Oil- Inspired by traditional Thai recipes for topical pain relief.

7 drops Plai + 4 drops Lime (or Makrut lime) + 4 drops peppermint essential oil + 3 drops Eucalyptus + 2 drops of Turmeric + 1 oz coconut oil (or Arnica Infused Oil)

Mood Boosting Diffuser Blend: 3 drops grapefruit + 2 drops of ylang ylang + 1 drop Plai

Safety

No known safety issues.

Rosemary *rosmarinus officinalis*

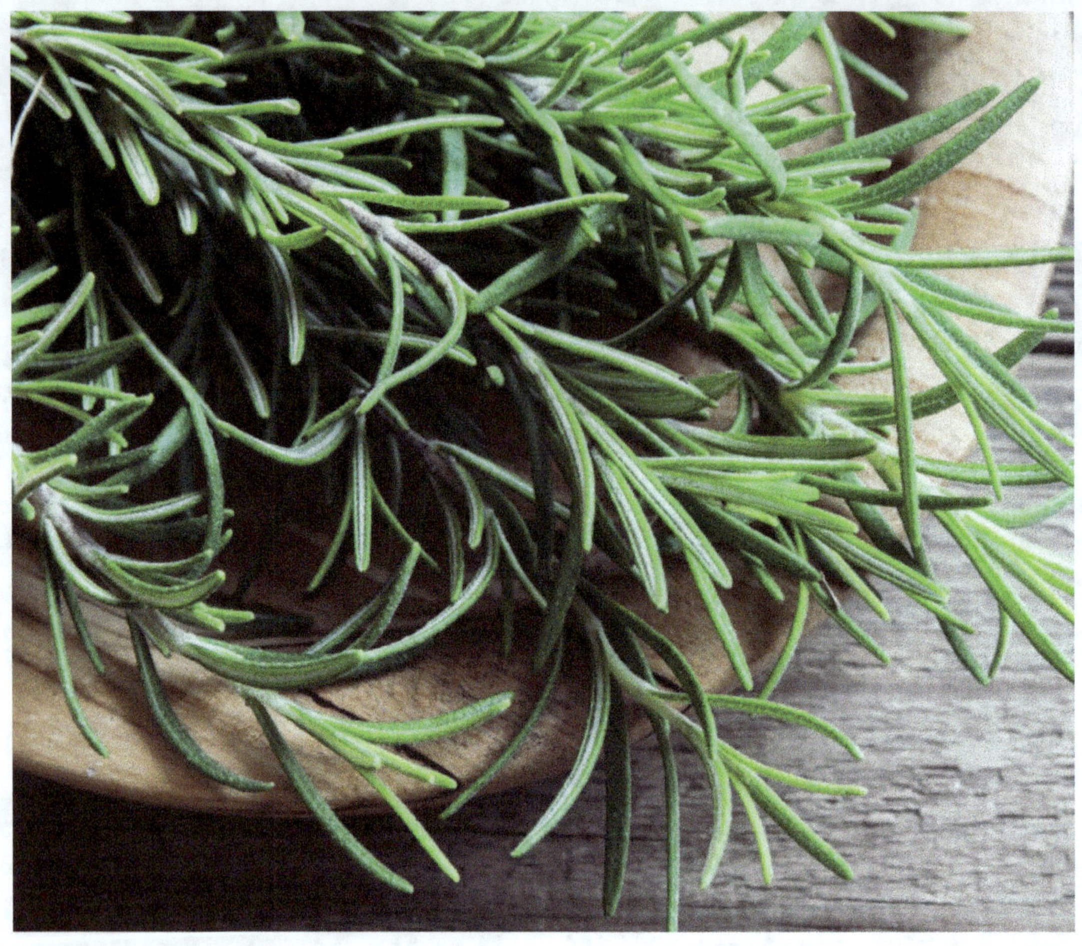

"Just as we learn how to start and not finish, we can learn to complete what we begin." – Sark

If Rosemary were human, she'd be the life of the party. She brings her creative power and juice everywhere she goes—and when she shows up in a space; you know it!

Rosemary has long been used to revitalize the senses, to cleanse the systems, and to clear the mind.

Its aroma is warm, herbaceous, camphorous-pine, and penetrating.

Background

Rosemary is an evergreen shrub that blooms pale blue blossoms from December through spring. It can grow close to 6 feet high. Its name means 'dew of the sea' because it naturally grows near the Mediterranean Sea.

For millennia, people have utilized this plant for medicinal purposes, and as a tradition, they burned its leaves to purify the air. They incorporated rosemary in Roman burial rites from ancient times until well into the middle ages, when it became customary to place branches of rosemary on the coffin during funerals. In medieval times Rosemary has been used in bouquets, symbolizing fidelity between marriage partners.

Main Constituents: Monoterpenes, Oxides, Ketones

Country of origin: Spain, Morocco, South Africa

Extraction Method: Steam distillation

Part of Plant used: Leaves

Therapeutics

Reduce mental and physical fatigue and sluggishness and stimulate your creative power! Long praised for its ability to support hair growth–rosemary is another extremely popular and versatile oil. It's enlivening, can awaken the mind, and works wonders on the joints and deep muscular tension.

Physical:

- Neuromuscular Pain
- Rheumatic pain - arthritic conditions
- Congested Skin, acne
- Muscle Relaxant- leg cramps, spasms
- Vein stimulant
- Warming
- Respiratory-Decongestant, expectorant, mucolytic
- Increases circulation
- Digestive
- Hair- growth, shine, luster
- Antioxidant

Emotional:

- Cephalic- brain tonic, aids memory
- Mental Clarity- brain fog
- Good for Lethargy or sluggishness
- Energizing
- Invigorating
- Creativity- frees mental restrictions
- Nervous system and general stimulant
- Restorative
- Oil of protection

Blends well with

Peppermint, Lavender, Basil, Lemon, Eucalyptus, Fir, Lemongrass, Pine, Tea tree, spice oils.

Bodyworker Applications

Mental Awakener: Bring vibrancy with this blend. Massage onto pulse points and inhale as needed. In a glass roller bottle mix: 2 drops Rosemary + 1 drops Basil + 2 drops Peppermint + 2 drops Lime + 10 ml Carrier oil

Overworked Muscles: 10-12 drops Rosemary essential oil + 1oz Carrier Oil

Scalp Conditioning Blend: Apply a small amount with a dropper, massage into scalp and hair, and leave overnight for a nourishing head treatment.

8 drops Rosemary essential oil + 4 drops Cedar essential oil + 4 drops Lavender essential oil + 4 drops Palmarosa essential oil + 4 drops Peppermint essential oil + 4 drops Lavender essential oil + 2 oz Argan, Almond or Jojoba Oil.

Safety

Possible skin sensitivity. Keep out of reach of children. If pregnant or under a doctor's care, consult your physician. Do not use undiluted on the skin, do not take internally.

Tea Tree *melaleuca alternifolia*

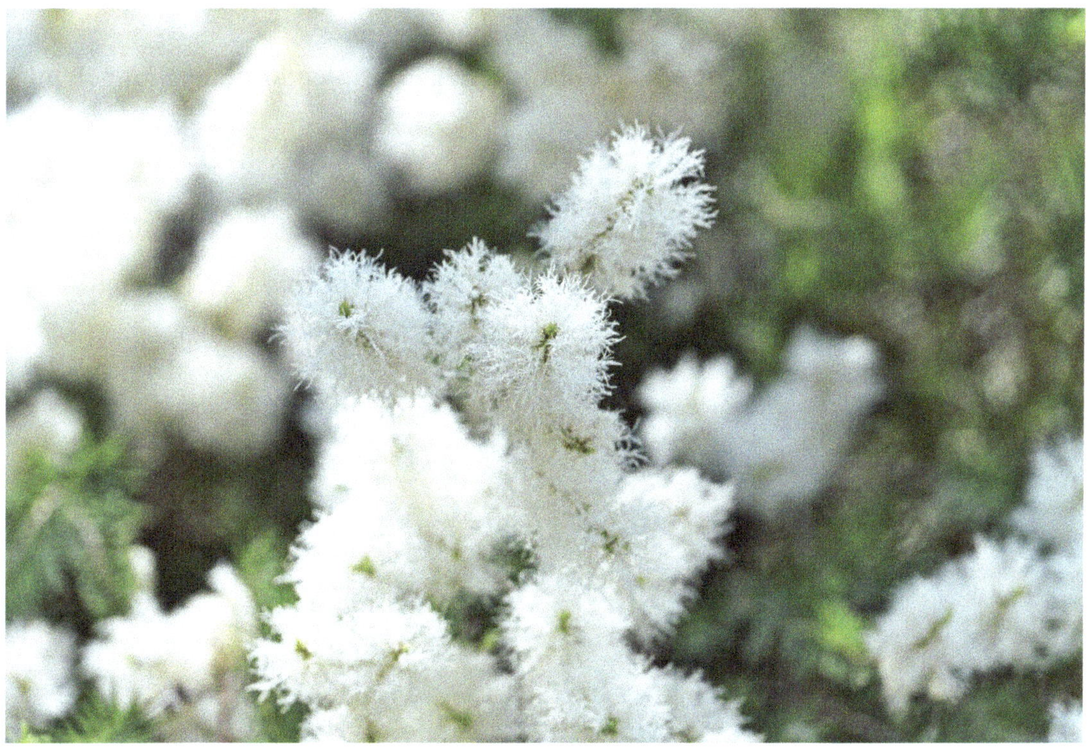

Tea Tree is a miracle worker for the skin– and helps treat wounds, bites, and fungal infections. This extremely versatile oil is a must have, and is great to make into a salve to support your clients with skin issues.

Its aroma is medicinal, fresh, camphorous, and herbaceous.

Background

Also known as Melaleuca, Tea tree essential oil has antiseptic properties, often used to help prevent infections. It was named by Captain Cook who brewed the tea for his sailors.

Because of its regenerative and cleansing properties, it has been used to help improve the skin, particularly with acne. "First Aid in a Bottle" is how many refer to Tea Tree because of its antifungal, antibacterial and antiseptic properties.

The Australian army used it as an antiseptic for wounds during World War II.

Main Constituents: Monoterpenes

Principal Places of Production: Australia

Part of Plant used: Leaves

Extraction method: Steam distillation

Therapeutics

A must have in your first aid kit! Anti-viral, anti-bacterial, anti-infectious, anti-fungal, purifying.

Physical:

- Achy Muscles and Joints
- Acne, oily skin
- Colds, flu
- Nail fungus
- Infected wounds
- Respiratory health

Emotional:

- Soothes mental stress
- Clears the mind
- Relieves anxiety and depression

Blends well with

Bergamot, Peppermint, Rosemary, Orange, Lavender, Eucalyptus, Lemongrass, Thyme essential oil.

Bodyworker Applications

Diffuse with your favorite oils to kill microbes in the air.

Freshen the Feet Spray: 10 drops of each of the following EO's: Peppermint + Tea Tree + Eucalyptus + 190 (95%) proof Alcohol + Purified water (or hydrosol of choice). Add your essential oils to a 4 oz PET of glass bottle with atomizer. Then add alcohol (fill bottle to 20-30% or more). Mix. Then add water.

Safety

Do not take tea tree oil internally. Do not apply directly to the eyes or mucous membranes. Keep away from dogs–tea tree is toxic to them.

Turmeric *curcuma longa*

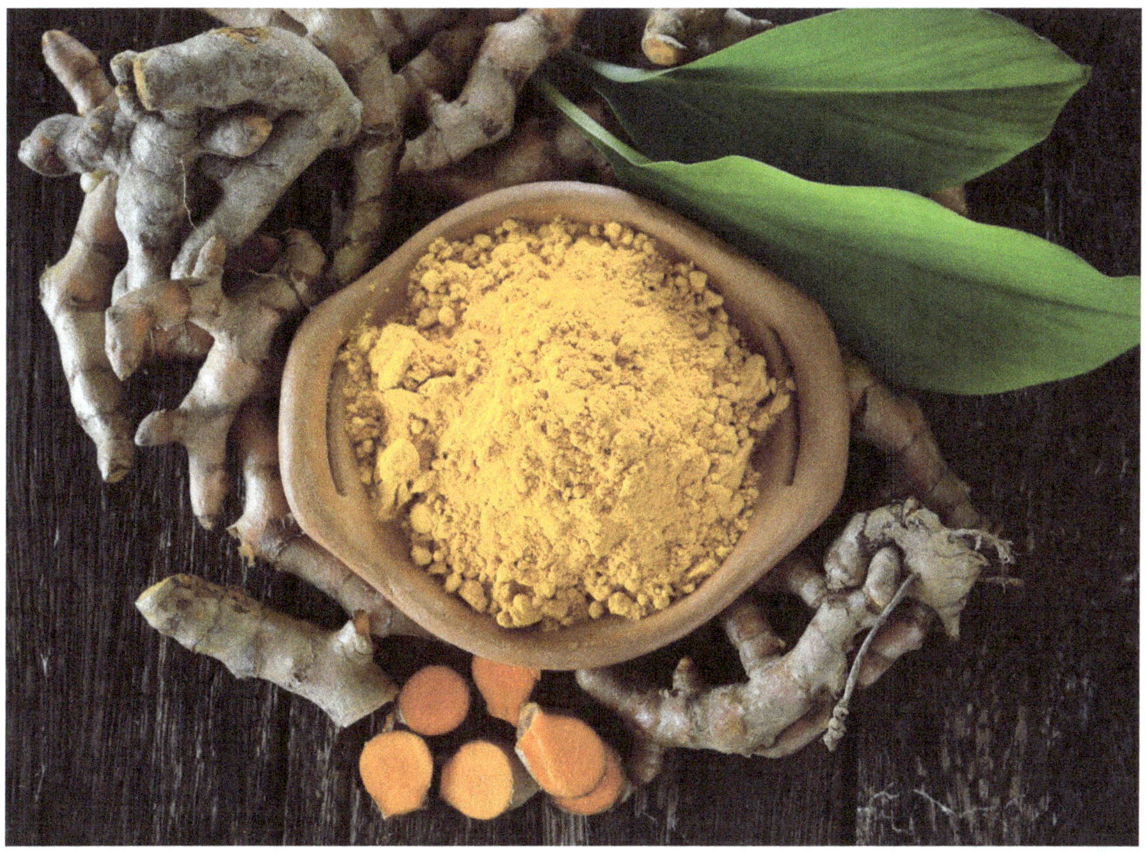

This vibrant herb has long been used to calm the nervous system, and is a great ally for healthy, glowing skin. Its aroma is warm, spicy, and exotic.

Background

Turmeric was referred to as "The Golden Goddess" by Ayurvedic healers in India over 5,000 years ago. In modern times, Turmeric has become a mainstream natural healing remedy.

The essential oil of Turmeric is found in the fleshy roots which are bright yellow-orange. Turmeric is a key ingredient in Indian cooking and is used in Ayurveda as an internal cleanser, especially for toning the kidneys and stimulating healthy digestion.

Main Constituents: Tumerones and sequineterpines

Principal Places of Production: India

Part of Plant used: Root

Extraction method: Steam Distillation

Therapeutics

Experience the therapeutic benefits of turmeric oil as its golden essence, sourced from the tropics, gently soothes and warms muscles and joints while nurturing skin health.

Physical:

- Anti-inflammatory
- Menstrual discomforts
- Joint pain- cold joints, rheumatism
- Skin blemishes
- Skin irritations
- Hair care
- Muscular Tension relief- neck, head, shoulders
- Warms the body- cold limbs
- Fixative- helps old aromas together

Emotional:

- Calms the nervous system
- Comforting
- Grounding
- Warmth

Blends well with

Spice oils such as Ginger, Black Pepper, Frankincense, Juniper, Orange, Lemon, Chamomile, peppermint.

Bodyworker Applications

Yellow Oil: 12 drops Turmeric + 10 drops Lavender + 4 drops Black Pepper or Ginger + 8 drops Peppermint + 2 oz carrier oil

Skin Toning: Cellulite, skin glow.

4 drops Turmeric + 2 drops Juniper + 4 drops Grapefruit + 1 oz Carrier oil

Safety

Non-toxic, non-irritating and non-sensitizing.

Vetiver *vetiveria zizanioides*

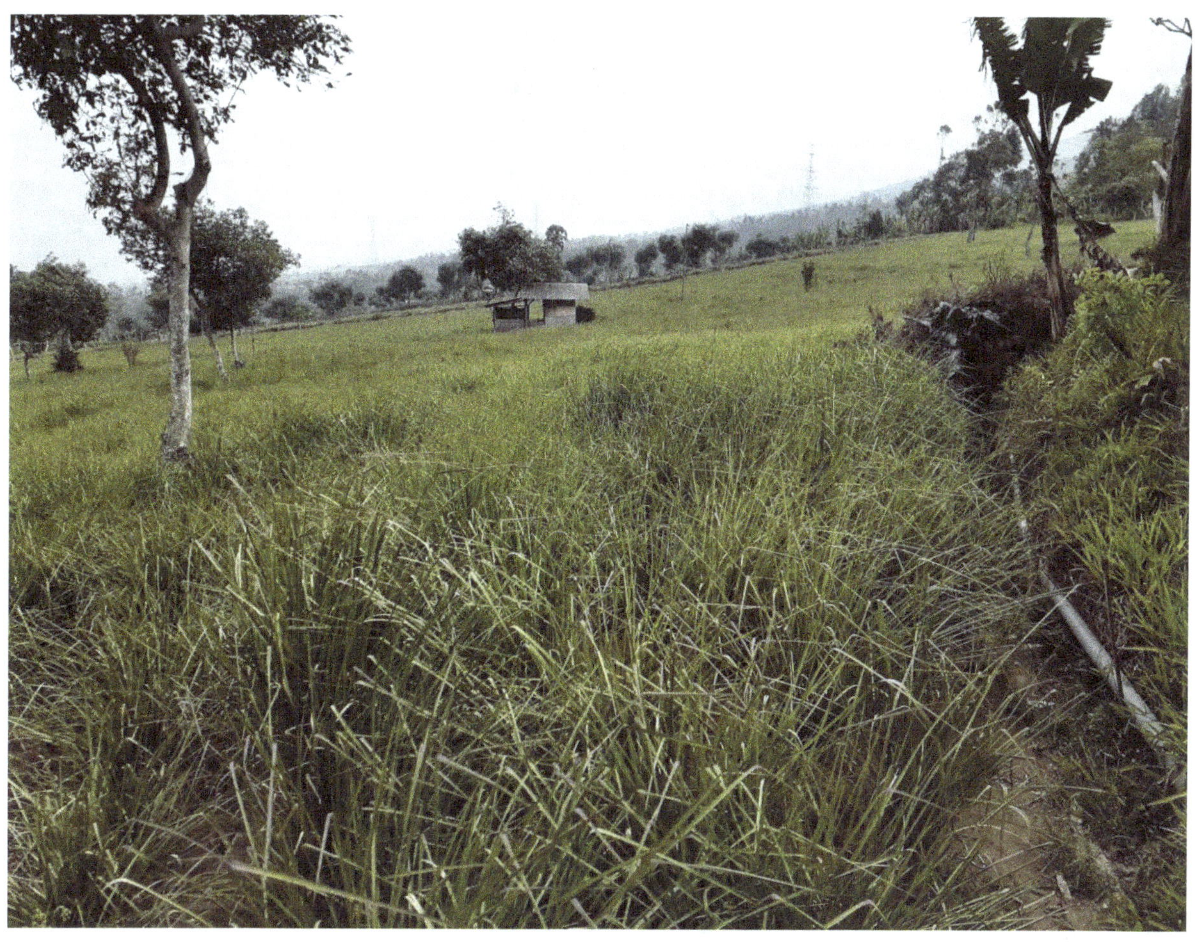

(Vetiver Field- Photo from Wild Harvest Indonesia)

A favorite in the perfume world, vetiver's scent is mesmerizing. It is a natural antioxidant that soothes inflammation and can help with joint stiffness and arthritis. Its aroma is deep and earthy.

Background

Vetiver belongs to the same botanical family as lemongrass and citronella. It is utilized to prevent soil erosion and regenerate damaged topsoils in marshlands. Oil from Vetiver grown in high altitudes may have a slightly different aromatic profile or chemical composition that is admired by many.

Its roots contain the earthy, warm and woody aroma of the soil. Its aromatic roots are the #1 fixative, about 90% in perfuming, (a base note used to hold the lighter top notes onto the skin).

Main Constituents: Alcohol-vetiverol

Principal Places of Production: Indonesia, Haiti

Part of Plant used: Root

Extraction method: Steam distillation

Therapeutics

Inhale the aroma of the cool soil and allow it to lift your stress away.

Physical:

- Muscle Spasms
- Cooling- heat stroke, fever
- "Hot", inflamed skin conditions
- Poor circulation
- Arthritis
- Stiffness
- Calms inflamed skin conditions- acne, or irritated skin.

Emotional:

- Stress-induced conditions-anything "stress related"
- Nervous tension
- Deeply Calming
- Anxiety
- Nervous exhaustion
- Difficulty "letting go" or "letting things be"
- Sleep aid
- Aphrodisiac
- Stabilizes- over-agitated mind
- Grounding

Blends well with

Lavender, Clary Sage, Palmarosa, Geranium, Bergamot, Sweet Orange, Mandarin, Cedarwood, Juniper, Yarrow, and Ylang Ylang.

Bodyworker Applications

Restore & Re-balance Blend: 4 drops Vetiver + 8 drops Geranium + 8 drops Clary Sage + 8 drops Lavender + 2 oz carrier oil.

Restless Anxiety Blend: 12 drops Cedarwood + 4 drops Juniper + 2 drops Vetiver + 1 oz carrier oil.

Rejuvenate the skin: Soothe and support hot, red or dry skin, add a drop of vetiver oil to your favorite chemical-free, unscented face or body cream or oil

Safety

Non-toxic, non-irritant and non-sensitizing. Use with caution during pregnancy (small amounts, diluted). Do not take vetiver essential oil internally.

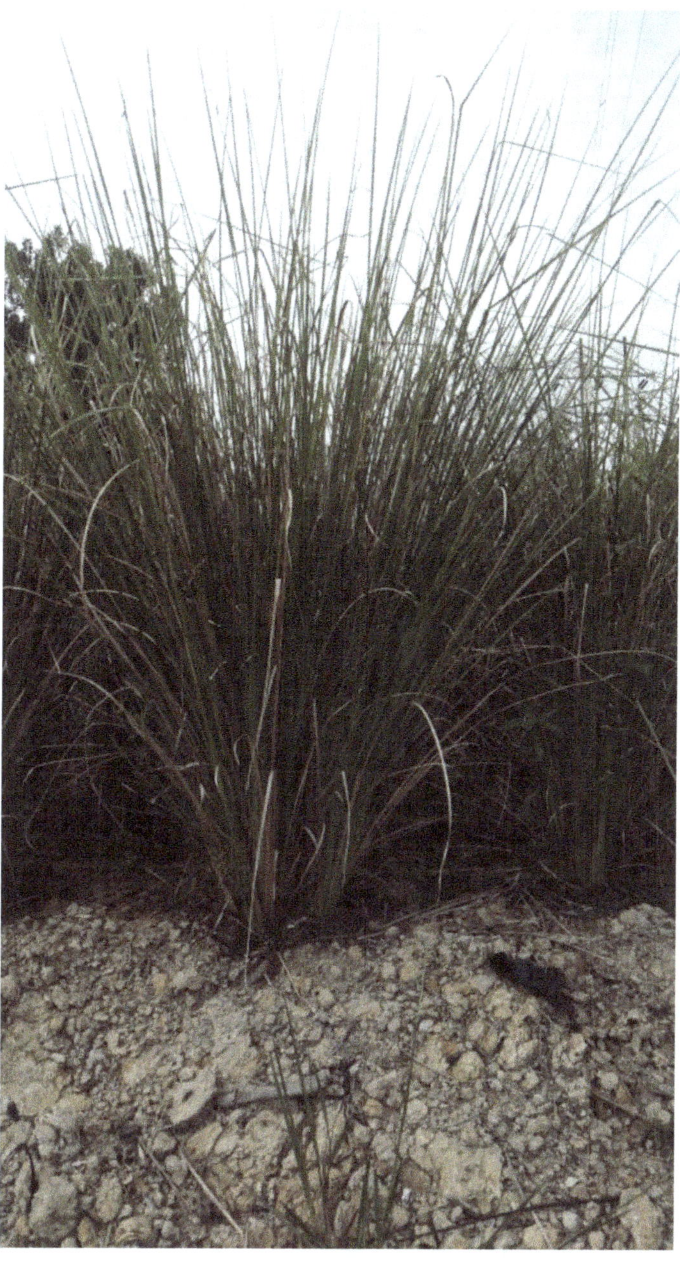

Vetiver Plant- Wild Harvest Indonesia

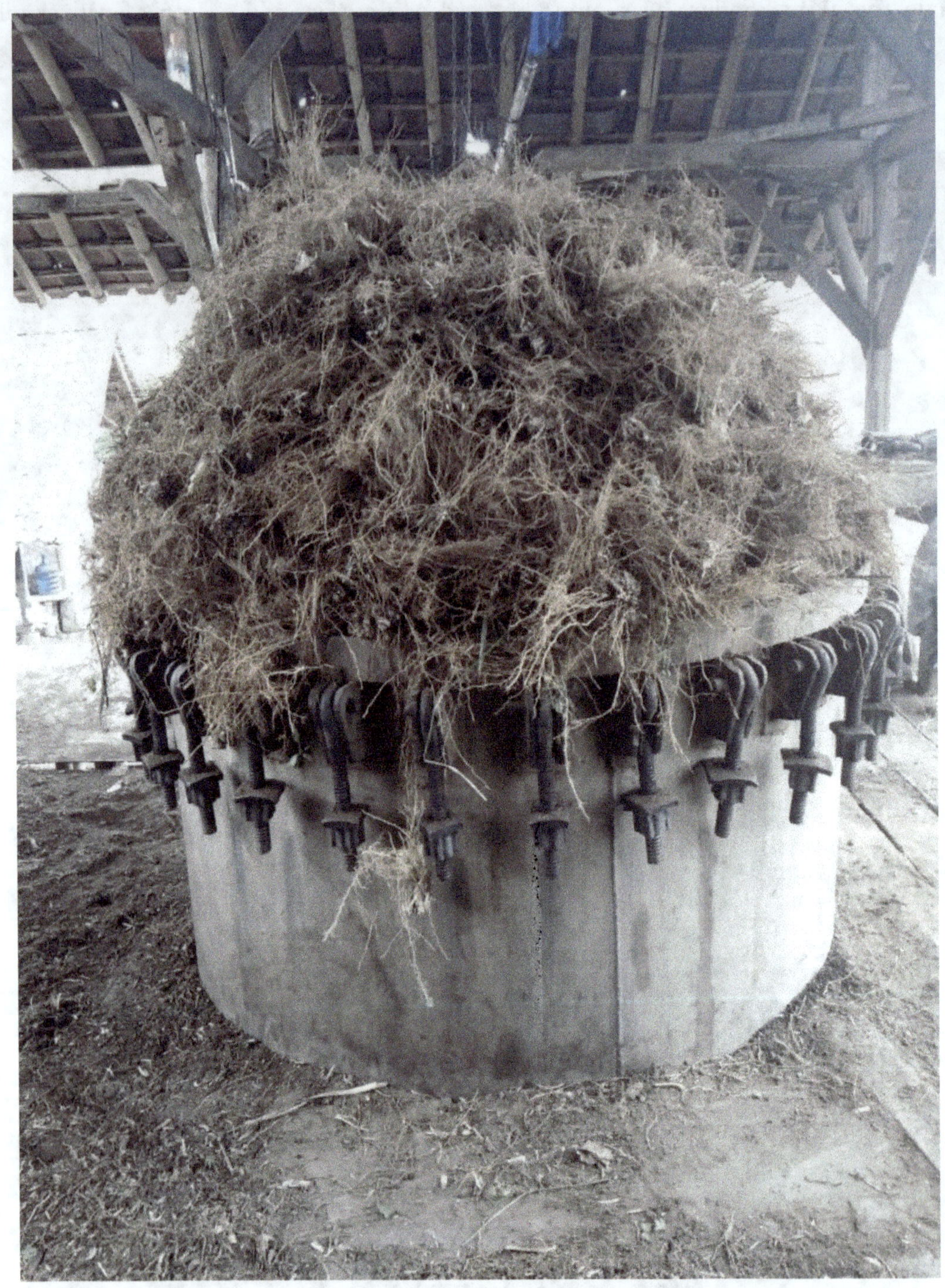

(Vetiver Distillation- Wild Harvest Indonesia)

Yarrow *Achillea millefolium*

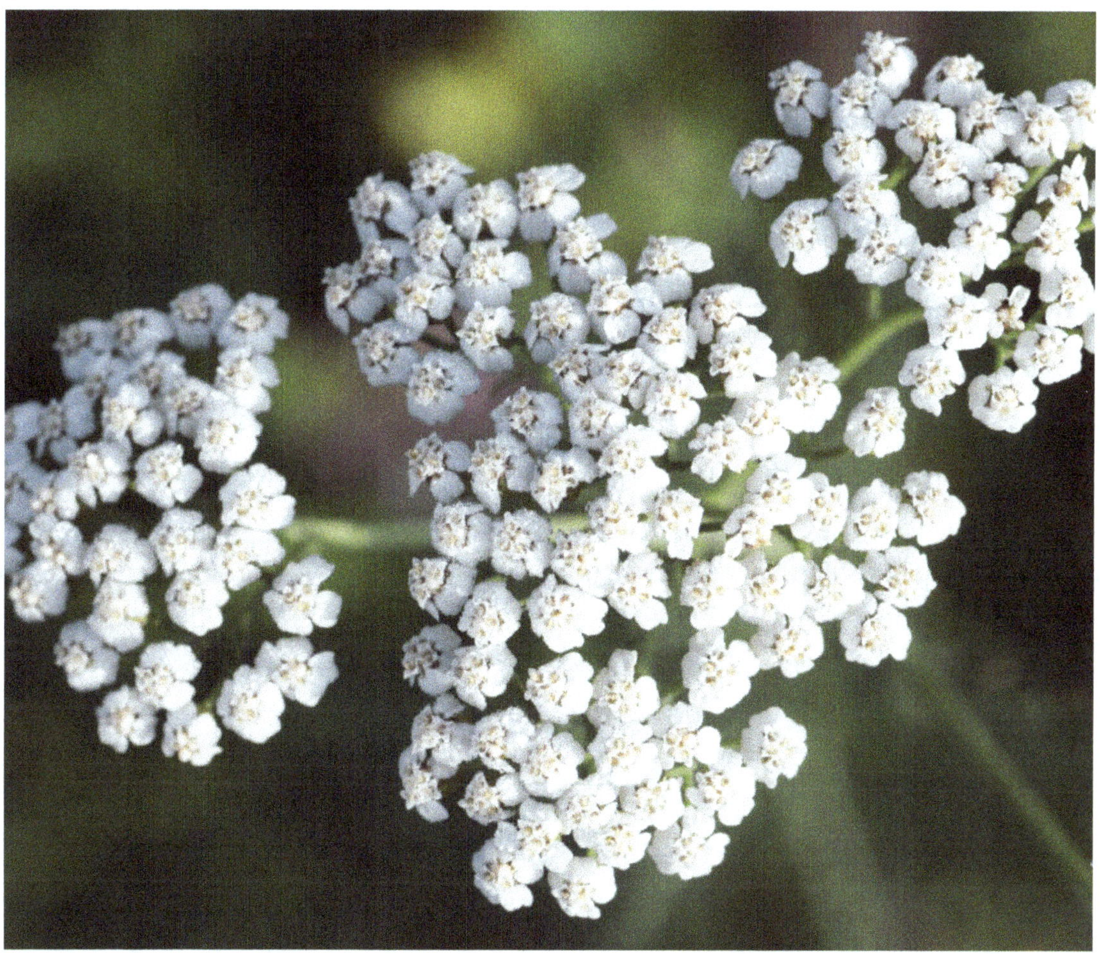

Yarrow, characterized by its robust, herbal, and sweet fragrance accompanied by a hint of camphor, presents itself as a blue essential oil boasting a versatile range of capabilities.

Background

Ancient civilizations revered yarrow, with its delicate white flowers and feathery leaves, for its myriad of medicinal properties. The Greeks called it "Achillea" after Achilles himself, while the Chinese referred to it as "hǎo" or "yáng wēn" meaning "good for everything." Herbalists have brewed yarrow infusions and poultices to treat everything from fevers and wounds to digestive issues and menstrual problems.

Fast forward to the present day, and yarrow continues to be valued for its medicinal benefits. Herbalists and natural health practitioners use yarrow for its anti-inflammatory, antiseptic, and astringent properties. Often applied topically, it accelerates wound healing, diminishes inflammation, and soothes skin irritations.

But Yarrow's healing powers don't stop there. Its essential oil, extracted from the plant's flowers and leaves, offers additional benefits for both the mind and body.

Yarrow is full of delightful smelling volatile oils, including the beautiful blue azulene. Its color can be clear to yellow, or light blue to deep rich blue.

Main Constituents: Monoterpenes, Sesquiterpenes

Country of origin: France, Bulgaria, Hungary, Germany, India

Extraction Method: Steam distillation

Part of Plant used: Leaves and Flowers

Therapeutics

Harnessing the therapeutic properties of yarrow essential oil can elevate the efficacy of healing salves, offering a gentle yet potent solution to soothe irritated skin and accelerate the healing process of minor cuts and scrapes. Its anti-inflammatory and analgesic qualities extend a comforting touch to sore muscles, while its calming effects on the nervous system provide a holistic approach to overall well-being.

Physical:

- Wound Care
- Rheumatism
- Arthritis
- Inflamed/Injured Muscles
- Muscular And Menstrual Cramps
- Scarring
- Acne
- Eczema
- Skin regenerative
- Hemorrhoids
- Digestive

Emotional:

- Introspection
- Emotional balance/stability
- Sedative
- Nervous Tension
- Meditative
- Antidepressant
- Stress-related conditions
- Promotes restful sleep
- Lifts the spirits

Blends well with

Bergamot, Bergamot mint, Lavender, Geranium, Clary Sage, Chamomile, Mandarin, Vetiver and cypress.

Bodyworker Applications

Tranquil Blue Massage oil: Deeply grounding, for balancing the nervous system.

5 drops Yarrow + 5 drops Mandarin + 3 drops Bergamot + 2 drops Vetiver + 1 oz carrier oil

Blue Dream Synergy Blend: To relieve insomnia caused by anxiety. Mix the following in an essential oil dropper bottle. Use in a diffuser, inhaler, roll-on, massage oil or in the bath.

1 ml Yarrow + 1 ml Lavender + 1 ml Roman Chamomile

Yarrow Tummy Soothe

Helps to expel intestinal gasses and reduces abdominal pain, gas pain, and flatulence. Massage in a clockwise motion.

8 drops Yarrow + 1 tbsp. Castor Oil or other carrier of choice.

Safety

According to Essential Oil Safety by Tisserand and Young (second edition), oils containing chamazulene could present a theoretical risk in that it could inhibit drugs metabolized by CYP1A3, CYP3A4 and CYP2D6 such as antidepressants, calcium channel blockers, and some chemotherapy drugs.

Ylang Ylang *cananga odorata*

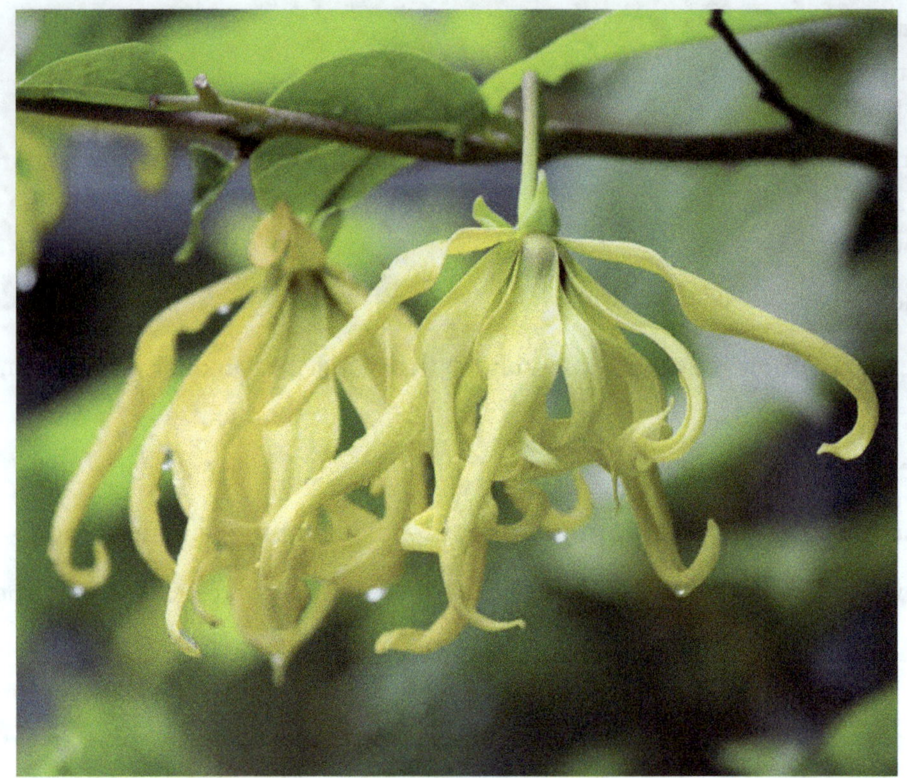

"The antidote to exhaustion is not (necessarily) rest. It's about wholeheartedness."
- David Whyte

The "flower of flowers." This exotic flower produces an intense perfume that deeply tranquilizes the body systems.

The potent aroma of ylang ylang, infused with spicy and musky undertones, is celebrated for its sensual and calming fragrance. It serves as a comforting essential oil and is also used to flavor beverages, candies, and even ice cream.

Background

Ylang Ylang Essential Oil is distilled from the flowers of a tall tropical tree that grows in Madagascar, China, Philippines, Indonesia and reunion islands. The name Ylang Ylang means "flowers of flowers".

Ylang Ylang is a beautiful oil. It is great for all skin types as it regulates sebum production in both mature and youthful skin. Additionally, it promotes the growth of fuller, more luxurious hair.

Everywhere Ylang Ylang grows, the flowers are a popular decoration, whether placed into the hair or woven into wreaths, or placed in rooms to fragrance the air.

In the Polynesian Islands, Ylang Ylang is mixed with coconut oil to create a fragrant blend used for massaging into the hair and body, offering both a pleasant scent and protective properties.

Ylang Ylang flowers are typically harvested early in the morning when their fragrance is most potent. The flowers are carefully hand-picked to avoid damaging them.

Note About Ylang Ylang Distillation:

In traditional distillation, Ylang Ylang essential oil is separated into different fractions or grades based on the boiling points of its components.

During the initial stages of distillation when the essential oil is first extracted from the Ylang Ylang flowers: Ylang Ylang Extra (Ylang Ylang I)

As the distillation process continues, additional fractions of essential oil are obtained, resulting in grades such as Ylang Ylang II. Finally, Ylang Ylang III is typically obtained towards the later stages of distillation when the remaining aromatic compounds are extracted from the Ylang Ylang flowers.

However, some producers opt for a different approach known as complete or full distillation. This distillation process is extended beyond the typical duration used for traditional Ylang Ylang essential oil production. This prolonged distillation allows for the extraction of a broader spectrum of aromatic compounds present in the Ylang Ylang flowers. Ylang Ylang Complete has a fuller and more rounded aroma compared to the individual grades obtained through fractional distillation. It may encompass a broader spectrum of fragrance notes, ranging from the intensely floral to deeper, earthier tones.

Ylang Ylang Complete is valued for its complexity and versatility, offering a more comprehensive representation of the Ylang Ylang flower's aromatic profile.

Main Constituents: Rich in sesquiterpenes, esters and alcohols.

Principal Places of Production: China, Philippines, Indonesia and reunion islands.

Part of Plant used: Flowers

Extraction method: Steam distillation

Therapeutics

Its floral aroma soothes the senses, calms the mind, and promotes deep relaxation, while its natural properties help to nourish and balance the skin and uplift the spirit.

Physical:

A study observed that Ylang Ylang has the potential to lower pulse rate and blood pressure, while simultaneously enhancing alertness and arousal.

- Scalp tonic- hair growth
- Skincare- stressed skin, oily or combination
- HBP-palpitations
- PMS - mood balancing, cramps
- Muscle cramping
- Eases physical discomforts- achy muscles
- Relaxes CNS
- Promotes restful sleep

Emotional:

Euphoric

- Aphrodisiac- balancing for both male and female
- Opens and expands the heart- inner trust
- Peace of mind
- Soothes and reduces anxiety, fear and anger
- Deeply calming
- Mood elevating-love
- Restorative nerve tonic
- Insomnia- aids deep sleep

Blends well with

Citrus oils such as Bergamot, Grapefruit, Orange, Lavender, Geranium, Clary Sage, and Vetiver.

Bodyworker Applications

Peaceful Massage Oil: Blend with carrier oil of your choice in 8 oz amber or cobalt PET Boston Round Bottle. 15 drops Ylang Ylang + 25 drops Lavender + 20 drops Cedarwood + 20 drops Orange

Balancing Face treatment: Apply with a dropper at night before bedtime on a clean face.

½ oz Jojoba Oil + ½ oz Almond Oil + 2 drops Ylang Ylang + 2 drops Geranium + 2 drops Frankincense

Luxurious Scalp Oil: 1 oz Sweet Almond or Argan oil + 5 drops Ylang Ylang + 2 drops Lavender

Balinese Massage Oil: 5 drops Ylang Ylang + 4 drops Vetiver + 3 drops Lemongrass + 1 oz fractionated coconut oil

Safety

Excessive use can cause headaches or nausea. Non-toxic, non-irritant and non-sensitizing. Do not take internally.

Self Care is for YOU too

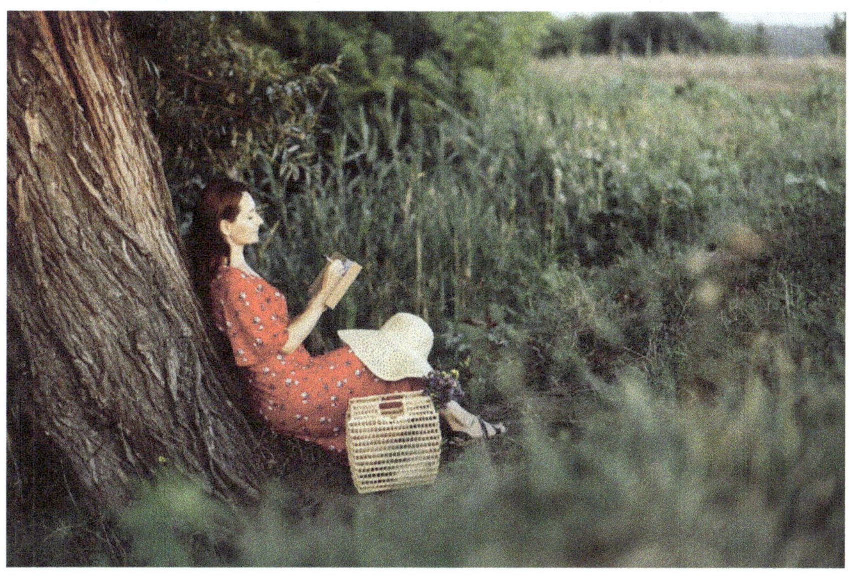

"Rest and self-care are so important. When you take time to replenish your spirit, it allows you to serve others from the overflow. You cannot serve others from an empty vessel."

Eleanor Brown

Let's talk about you. It's in our nature as bodyworkers to give, give, and give some more to our clients. We genuinely want them to feel better, and we want to show and teach them how to take tender care of themselves, too.

But are we taking our own medicine?

I've seen more colleagues than I'd like to count face burnout within the first few years of their practice–and it has a lot to do with neglecting their own self care.

We can only serve our clients to the capacity that we serve ourselves. You've heard it–we can't pour from an empty cup, and we shouldn't try to. When you practice self-care regularly, the way you show up in your practice and in your life transforms.

Your clients will be more inspired to follow because you are leading by example. When we find that we have a pattern of clients that are unwilling to take charge of their wellbeing, ask yourself, are you doing it?

In the realm of self-care, it's crucial to recognize that aromatic oils act as allies rather than sole agents of change. While they provide invaluable support, they serve as companions on our journey inward, guiding us to unearth the roots of our challenges. Understanding the essence of our struggles is essential for true transformation. Thus, active engagement is paramount; it is through our deliberate participation that meaningful shifts occur. Embrace your role as an active participant in your well-being journey, for it is through your conscious efforts that lasting change blossoms.

Self-care looks different for everyone, and it's important to listen to your intuition and do what feels best for you and your body. Here are some ways you can incorporate self-care using the power of Aromatherapy.

These recommendations are for both you and your clients. But they're for you, first.

Aromatherapy Bath

We all know a nice, long bath with a candle and soothing music works wonders, especially on our bodies that go through so much. Incorporating a luxurious soak a few times a week is a great way to recover and to relax. Create your own home sanctuary and work your new expanded knowledge of essential oils into the mix.

Abhyanga Self Massage

Abhyanga, the Sanskrit word for massage, is an important part of Ayurvedic wellness and you can perform it on yourself to restore balance and energy. It can help relieve aches and pains, soften and tone the skin, relax nervous tension, and increase circulation.

Carve out 20-30 minutes, grab some oil, and take your time. Massage your head and temples, chest, arms, belly, hips, legs, and feet. You can warm the oil by placing the bottle in a bowl of warm water to add an extra touch. Your body will thank you.

You can also teach your clients this to use as a self-care ritual in between sessions. Typically, Abhyanga is performed in the morning before a shower or bath, but fit it in when you can.

Sesame oil is a common choice for its warming properties, while coconut oil is known for its cooling effects, and Jojoba oil is used to maintain balance.

A Cup of Tea

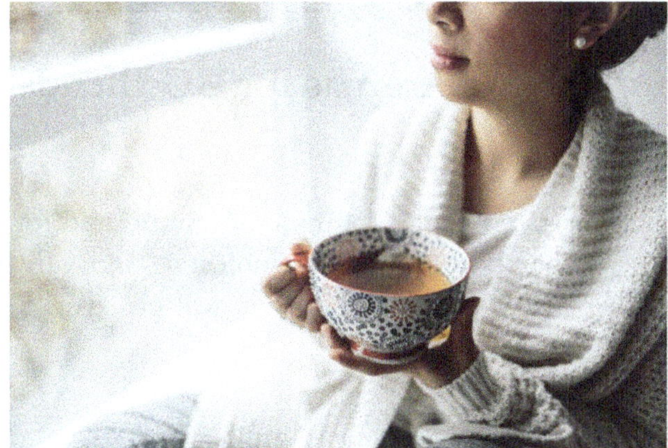

A cup of tea is sometimes all you need to reset. Self-care does not have to be a time intensive thing.

Pausing for a moment and having a cup of your favorite herbal tea while diffusing your favorite essential oil can make a huge impact on your state of being. Relax your mind, gather your thoughts, and just *be* for a minute.

Our nervous system is our connection between our inner and outer worlds. We need to nourish it, giving it proper care so that it can replenish and support us through the different cycles of our life.

We want to avoid abusing or overtaxing this important system so that we don't suffer emotional and physical burnout, where our thirst for life becomes flat and spiritless.

Aromatherapy massage and herbal interventions work beautifully to support us from the inside out.

Here are some herbs that support a healthy nervous system and are especially great to keep at hand during times of stress. You can find them available from an herb supplier to make an infusion or purchase as a tincture:

- Chamomile
- Lemon balm
- Linden
- St. John's wort
- Valerian
- Passion flower
- Green Tea
- Rooibos

Journal prompt: How will you incorporate self-care for yourself? What would you recommend to your clients?

A Note on Aromas for EO Blends

In aromatherapy, terms such as top, middle, and base notes are used to categorize essential oils by their aromas and rates of evaporation. Notes are subjective and vary from book to book, and depending on which aromatherapist you talk to, but this will give you a good starting point when creating your own blends.

A balanced blend has a mixture of these 3 notes:

Top Notes

Top notes evaporate rapidly and give the initial impact of a blend.

Examples of top notes: Bergamot, Eucalyptus, Basil, Grapefruit, Lavender, Lemon, Lemongrass, Lime, Mandarin, Orange, Peppermint, and Spearmint.

Middle Notes

Middle notes bring the blend together. They give the body to the blend and have harmonizing effects. The middle notes become noticeable after a few minutes of inhaling the aroma. Most are soft and subtle.

Examples of middle notes: Basil, Bay Laurel, Carrot Seed, Chamomile, Cinnamon, Clary Sage, Cypress, Fennel, Geranium, Jasmine, Marjoram, Neroli, Palmarosa, Rose, Rosemary, Rosewood, Spruce, Tea Tree, Thyme, and Ylang Ylang.

Base Notes

These are your rich, heavy scents. They solidify the blend and slow the evaporation of the other oils (fixatives). Their deep aromas usually linger as they evaporate slowly. Many of them come from woods, resins and roots.

Examples of base notes: Cedarwood, Frankincense, Ginger, Myrrh, Patchouli, Sandalwood, Turmeric, and Vetiver.

EO Scent Categories

Throughout the day, closely observe how various scents affect your mood, both positively and negatively. Actively seek scents that uplift you, whether it's the aroma of terpenes wafting from conifer trees, the scent of freshly baked cookies, or the familiar fragrance of your favorite soap or perfume. When facing emotional challenges, deliberately surround yourself with these comforting aromas and observe how they influence your mood.

In the realm of aromatherapy, individuals often find themselves drawn to specific categories of aromas. When encountering an essential oil or blend, take a moment to analyze its scent and consider what aspects you find appealing or unappealing. Are there particular aroma categories that consistently resonate with you more than others?

Aromatic Families

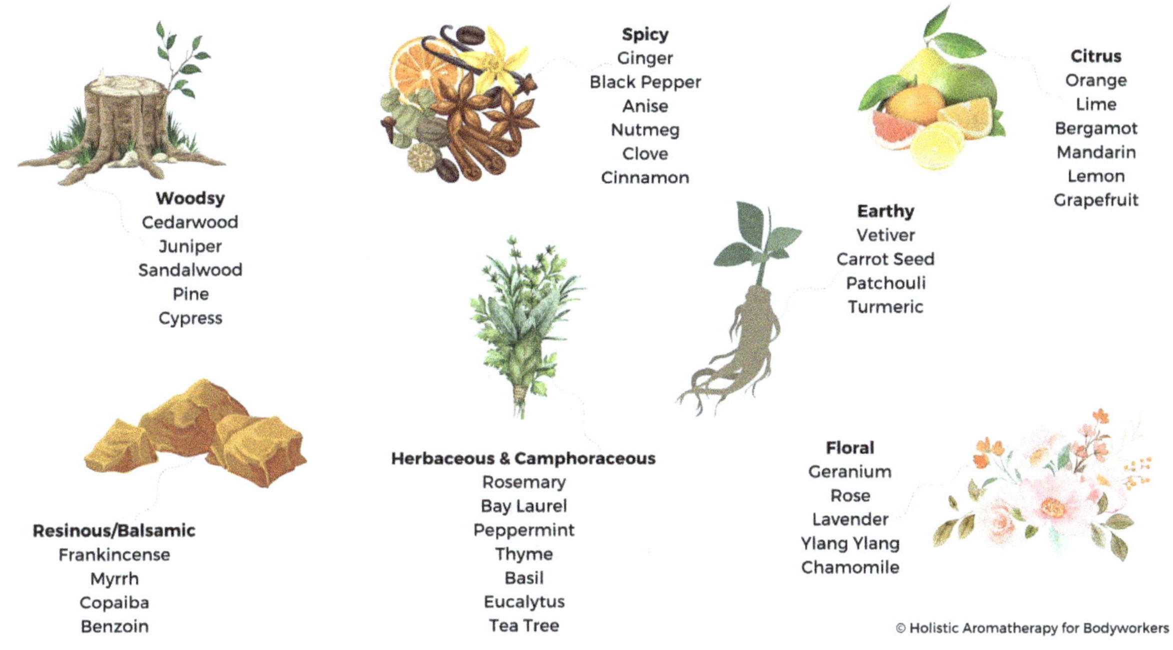

© Holistic Aromatherapy for Bodyworkers

Blending Basics

There is beauty in simplification when making your own blends. You can create powerful blends with just a few oils.

Creating a Synergy

A synergy is the cocktail generally made up of 3–5 essential oils that are blended together for an individual based on their specific goals. A well-balanced synergy contains oils that support each other to help balance the body and mind.

First, listen to your clients. What are they saying? What is their body language like? Did they tell you a story? What are their concerns? How are their condition/symptoms manifesting physically and emotionally? Do I focus my blend on the physiological or emotional manifestations, or both?

The pyramid method: Use this guideline to help you create your synergy.

1. **Primary/specific:** With the information you collected from your clients above, we can choose the "primary" essential oil with the intention of targeting the primary goal(s) for the recipient. This will be the base or root of the formula. What oils come to mind? Why? Take notes.
2. **Supporters:** Then, choose additional oils to support these goals. These oils can be adaptogens that will enhance and harmonize your blend. (1-2 oils)
3. **Activators/catalyst:** These oils give life to your blend. They are the movers and the shakers. What oils come to mind promoting movement and energize the blend (cleansing, stimulating, warming, and energizing herbs)?

Once you create your synergy, determine the most beneficial applications, such as massage oil, cream, bath salt, inhaler, etc. massage oil, cream, bath salt, inhaler, ect.

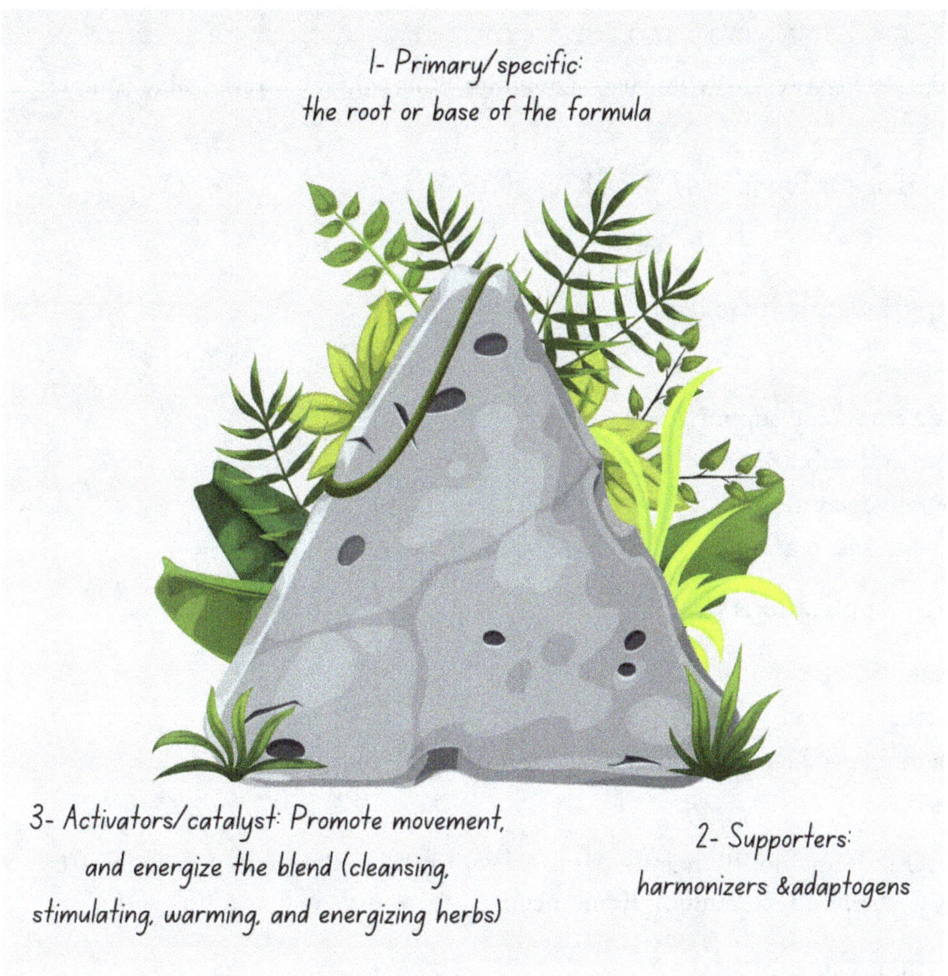

Example: Blending for the Physiological Approach

Varicose Veins

Aromatherapy Treatment Goals:

- Reduce Pain
- Enhance circulation
- Prevent varicose veins from getting worse
- Support and strengthen the veins
- Reduce pain

Aromatherapy Applications:

- Gel
- Massage Oil

Beneficial EO's: Cypress, Rosemary, Lavender, Geranium, Grapefruit, Juniper, Frankincense, Lemongrass, Lime.

Example: Blending for Emotional/Mental Support

Anxiety

Aromatherapy Treatment Goals:

- Reduce stress
- Provide emotional support
- Ground and stabilize
- Encourage relaxation
- Reduce muscle tension

Aromatherapy Applications

- Massage
- Aromatherapy Baths
- Inhalation: create customized inhaler for individual to use as needed
- Diffusion

Beneficial EO's: Bergamot, Bergamot Mint, Sweet Orange, Mandarin, Lavender, Clary Sage, Vetiver, Ylang Ylang, Cedarwood, Geranium, Frankincense.

Aromatherapy Case Studies

The following real life case studies serve as examples of aromatherapy applications.

Case Study: Neuroma Surgery

In this real-life aromatherapy case study, the client underwent surgical removal of a large neuroma, which had been affecting a nerve and causing pain and numbness in the index finger. Significant swelling was present, along with numbness and hypersensitivity to touch, post-surgery.

The aromatherapy treatment aimed at alleviating nerve pain, hypersensitivity, and swelling, with the primary goals being analgesia and reducing inflammation. The custom blend consisted of Arnica Infused Oil (50%) and Almond Oil (50%), combined with essential oils including Frankincense, Lavender, German Chamomile, Copaiba, and Birch.

The blend was applied distally over the thenar region and index finger as often as needed until the removal of stitches. Additionally, gentle cross-fiber massage was recommended over the closed incision after the wound healed.

The patient reported significant pain relief after using the oil, reducing pain levels from an 8-9 to a 1-2, without the need for over-the-counter painkillers except for the first day post-surgery. This successful outcome highlights the efficacy of aromatherapy in managing post-operative pain and promoting comfort during the healing process.

Case Study: Apendectomy

In this case study, the client underwent an emergency appendectomy, during which the surgeon encountered difficulties leading to larger-than-usual incisions. Following the surgery, the client requires aromatherapy support to aid in recovery from the traumatic procedure and facilitate a smoother healing process.

The primary goals of the aromatherapy blend are to relieve pain, reduce bruising and inflammation, minimize scar tissue formation, and promote overall healing. The formula consists of a massage oil with a 5% dilution, combining Jojoba Oil with therapeutic essential oils including Frankincense, Lavender, Helichrysum Itallicum, and Vitamin E.

This customized blend is designed to provide targeted relief and support, addressing both physical discomfort and the aesthetic aspects of scar reduction. By incorporating high-quality essential oils known for their anti-inflammatory, analgesic, and skin-regenerating properties, the aromatherapy formula aims to optimize the client's post-operative recovery experience, promoting comfort and facilitating the healing process.

Case Study: Muscular Pain & Stress/Tension (combination approach)

In this case study, the client, who receives massage therapy every 6-8 weeks due to a demanding work travel schedule, presents with chronic muscular tension and pain, particularly in the neck and shoulders, alongside high levels of stress and mental fatigue.

The treatment goals for aromatherapy focus on reducing muscular tension and pain, improving circulation, reducing stress, and providing a sense of breathing space. Considering the client's travel schedule, convenience and compliance with home use are essential factors.

The aromatherapy application involves a 90-minute aromatherapy massage session with a custom formula, incorporating techniques such as cupping and Gua Sha. The custom formula includes Cypress, Eucalyptus, Lavender, and Black Pepper essential oils. To ensure continued relief during travel, the client is provided with a roll-on containing the same formula.

During the follow-up, the client reports significant improvement, noting that the roll-on effectively alleviates tension in the neck and trapezius muscles. Moreover, the client finds the aroma therapy extremely relaxing during stressful periods, providing relief from a different kind of tension. Overall, the client expresses gratitude for the holistic approach to managing both physical and mental well-being.

Creating your Synergy Worksheet

What is your INTENTION or GOAL(s)?

____

____

____

What is your main FOCUS?

____

____

____

What essential oils come to mind to achieve these goal(s) and why?

____

____

____

Your Synergy:

1. **Primary/specific essential oil:**
2. **Supporters:**
3. **Activators/catalyst:**

My blend:

____

____

____

____

____

Making Synergies for Larger Quantities

For larger batches, use the following method instead of the one-drop-at-a-time method. This keeps your synergy all in one bottle that you can use to make your oils, butters, sugar scrubs, inhalers, etc.

You will need a graduated cylinder (that measures in ml) and a few droppers. Using a graduated cylinder, 1 ml equals approximately 25 drops. (See Measurements and Dilutions pg.200)

Synergy for a Good Night's Sleep

You will need a small graduated cylinder and third that measures by the milliliter.

In your graduated cylinder, add the following Essential Oils:

- 1 ml Lavender–nervine, comforting, promotes feelings of security, reduces agitation.
- 1 ml Mandarin - calming to the nervous system, uplifting, balancing.
- 2 ml Bergamot - balancing, calms anxious feelings.
- 1 ml Vetiver- grounding, cooling, promotes deep relaxation, restorative.

You now have your synergy. This makes a perfect blend for an inhaler, or diffuser. You can use this method as a formulation to create synergies that are ready to use and dilute appropriately for the treatment or product you create.

How do they smell together?

Once you've chosen your oils, see how they smell blended together. To avoid waste by creating a product that you don't like, add a drop of each oil to a cotton ball to see what the blend will smell like. You can also open the bottles together and circle them under your nose.

If there is oil you want to replace or remove–now's the time. And if you're happy with your synergy, you can now make your formula or product.

Blending Tips & Tricks

- Blend with intent. Don't just mix stuff together.
- Less is more- start by adding one drop at a time. You can add more to a blend, but you can't take away from it. Try adding a few drops to a piece of tissue to see if you like the combination first.
- Use combinations of top, middle and base notes for a well-balanced formula.
- Take notes! Document your recipes in a journal so that you can recreate the ones you love. Document what didn't work too.
- Blend oils with similar properties (Energizing, calming, relaxing, etc.)
- Add "lightness" to a heavy formulation with citrus notes.
- Listen to your clients- What are their needs? Take a proper health history and ask good questions.
- When creating a blend for someone else, provide them with clear directions and ingredients.
- Label your products with ingredients, date and store away from heat and sunlight.

Making Massage & Body Oils

If nothing else, one skill I hope you put to use after reading this book is to make your own massage oils! It's fun, incredibly easy–and will be a total wow factor when you blend it on the spot for your clients.

Step 1: Choose your carrier oil(s)

Play around a bit to get to know your perfect carrier oil blend - one that moves and feels like you want it to.

Step 2: Choose your essential oils or blend from one of the recipes in the profiles section.

Step 3: Add your essential oils to the glass bottle first, then add your carrier oil(s). Cover and shake gently. Your blend is ready to use. Do note that you won't be able to capture the full aromatic profile right away; massage oil formulations smell best after they are allowed to sit for about 24 hours. This allows all the molecules to disperse.

Bottle, and massage away!

Making your own facial massage oil

- Use gentle carrier oils for the face such as **Jojoba, Apricot, Camellia, Grape Seed and Argan oil.**
- Dilute at .5-1% max for the facial region

Sample Facial Massage Combinations:

Baby Skin: A gentle oil for all skin types, especially sensitive skin. 1 oz Apricot or Jojoba oil + 3 drops Lavender + 3 drops Roman Chamomile

Skin Balance: Excellent for dry, mature skin. Argan or Almond Oil + 2 drops Geranium + 2 drops Frankincense + 2 drops Lavender

Skin Revitalize: A restorative blend beneficial for oily or combination skin. 1 oz Apricot or Jojoba oil + 2 drops Copaiba Balsam + 1 drop Tea Tree + 1 drop Palmarosa + 1 drop Ho wood + 1 drop Lavender

Restorative Aromatherapy Facial Massage Sequence

A rejuvenating aromatherapy facial massage sequence designed to soothe the senses and revitalize the skin.

1. Begin at the bridge of the nose, between the eyes, at the bottom of the forehead. Using both thumbs, one following the other stroke in a continuous line up to the center toward the hairline.
2. Glide across the forehead, using all of the fingers of both hands from the center of the forehead toward the temples.
3. Place both hands on the forehead. Hold for a count of 10.
4. Press under eyebrows outward.
5. Press outer corner of the eyes.
6. Starting at the corners of the nose, with both hands work outward towards the ear. Repeat the movement outward until you cover the entire cheek and reach the corner of the mouth.
7. Use two fingers to glide outward between the nose and upper lip, then under the lower lip. Repeat several times. Pinch gently along the jawline, working outwards.
8. Press along the hairline from the center working towards the temples. Repeat several times.
9. Final Sweeps using both hands over both sides of the face, over the forehead, up both sides of the neck, and into a classic shoulder and neck glide to finish.

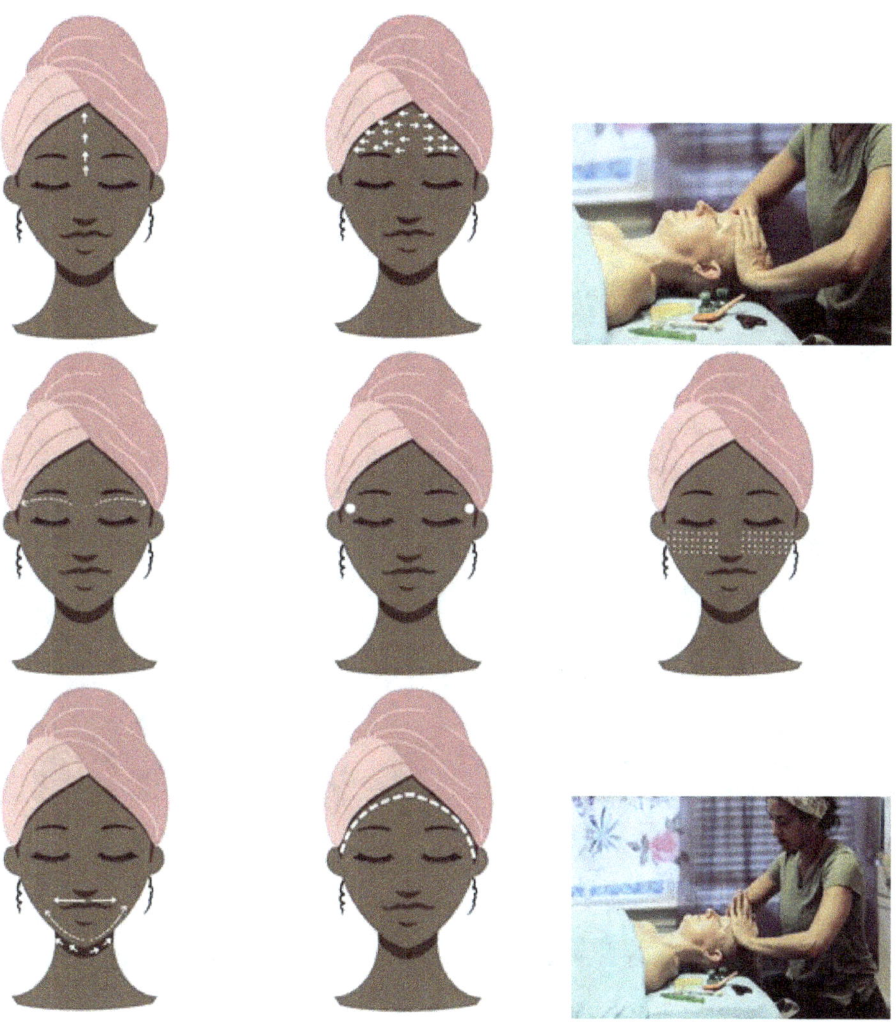

Aromatic Spa Treatments

Aromatic Spritzers:

Add EO's first to a 4 oz glass, PET plastic or aluminum bottle with atomizer. Then add 190 (95%) proof alcohol. Mix. Then add water, or your favorite hydrosol.

Fill the bottle with a minimum of 20-30% 150 Proof Alcohol (such as ever clear), then the remaining with water. When using solubol instead of alcohol, it is recommended to use a ratio of 1 part essential oil to 4 parts solubol.

1. Facial mist 8-10 drops of essential oils per 4 oz.
2. Body spray 30-40 drops per 4 oz.
3. Room spray 80-100 drops per 4 oz.

Exfoliating Scrubs

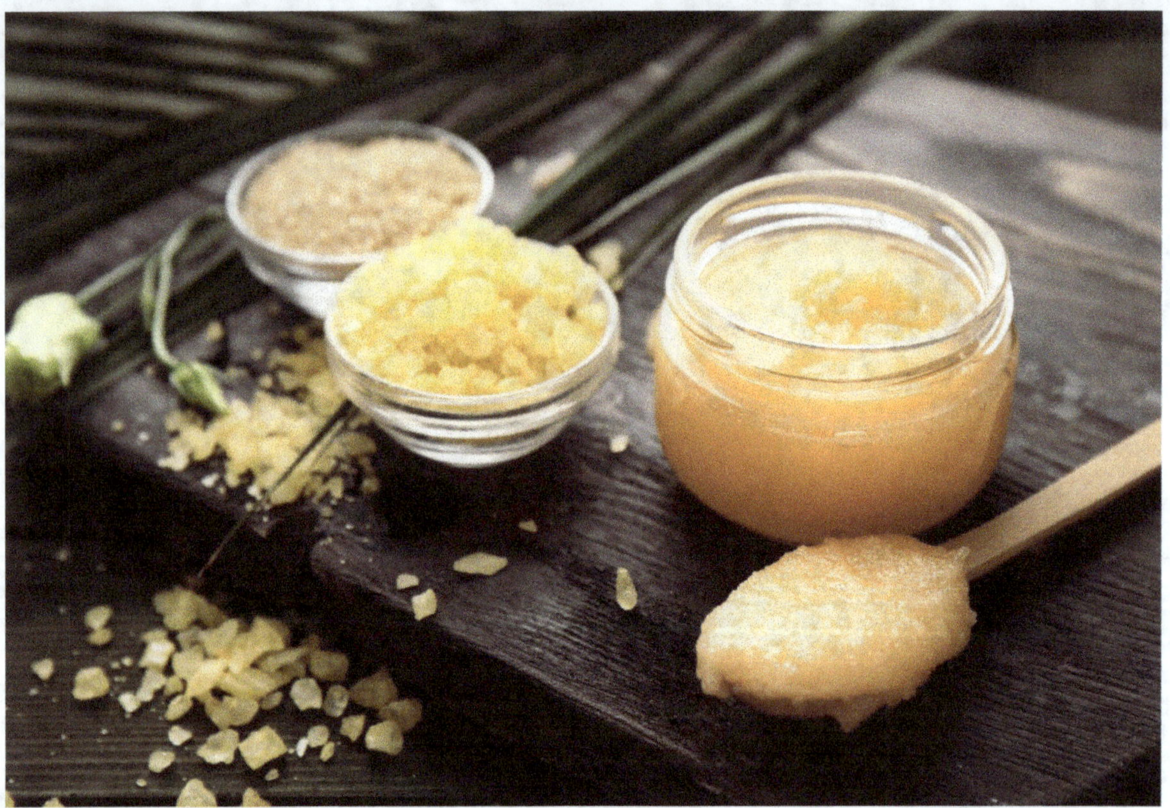

The following recipes are for use on the body; Not for use on the face. Use on clean skin. Do not use after shaving or on irritated skin. May leave a film of oil on your shower floor. Make sure to clean to avoid slipping!

Adjust the amount of carrier oil depending how wet or dry you prefer your scrub. Blend all of the ingredients together in a PET plastic jar.

Simple Sugar Scrub Recipe

- 8oz Raw can sugar
- 4 oz Carrier oil (I like to use lighter carrier oils for scrubs such as fractionated coconut or apricot)
- 10-15 drops Essential Oils
- Coffee Scrub
- ½ cup Coffee grounds
- ½ cup Raw cane sugar
- ¼-½ cup Sweet almond oil
- 5 drops Nutmeg
- 10 drops Sweet Orange

Green Earth Foot Scrub

- ½ cup Avocado Oil
- ¼ cup Fine Himalayan salt (or sea salt)
- 5 drops Cedarwood
- 5 drops Vetiver
- 5 drops Bergamot

Cabana boy sugar scrub:

- 8 oz Raw can sugar
- 4 oz Fractionated coconut oil
- 3 drops Lime
- 5 drops Palmarosa
- 5 drops Grapefruit
- 2 drops Lemongrass
- 2 drops Vetiver

Creamy Sugar Scrub

With a handheld mixer, whip the shea butter and oils together to desired consistency. Add sugar and whip until fully blended. You may add more oil if desired, or castor oil for a "stickier" consistency.

- 2.5 oz Virgin Coconut Oil
- 4.5 oz Shea Butter
- 1.5-2 oz Almond oil (or other carrier oil)
- 12 oz Raw cane sugar

Foot Baths

Aromatics can be added to a foot bath before a massage or reflexology treatment. Not only will this prep your clients' feet by softening rough skin, it will also prep them mentally, allowing them to get grounded and ready to receive.

For a simple foot bath, mix a handful of Epsom salt + 3-5 drops essential oil + 1 tbsp. Castile soap.

Saunas

If you have a sauna in your practice, you can enhance the sauna experience with essential oils.

Just place a bowl with hot water and essential oils in the corner of the cabin, and voila!

SAFETY PRECAUTION: Essential oils are flammable- do not place near a direct heat source or on any electrical appliances!

For the following recipes, blend your oils first in a bottle. Then add 10 drops of essential oil per 3 cups of water in your bowl.

Relaxing Sauna

- 10 drops cedarwood
- 5 drops Bergamot
- 2 drops Palmarosa

Invigorating Sauna

- 4 drops Scotch Pine
- 3 drops Rosemary
- 2 drops Eucalyptus*
- 7 drops Lime

*Eucalyptus used singly or combined also makes a fantastic addition to a sauna and can help clear the respiratory tract and clear the head.

Body polishes or exfoliations are offered at most spas. But you can easily create your own formulas in house. You can easily infuse mud wraps with essential oils and hydrosols as well.

Warm Embrace Cocoon

Product:

- 2 oz Sweet almond oil, or butter
- 4 drops Ginger
- 8 drops Sweet Orange
- 4 drops Black Pepper

If you prefer butter as your base, the soft butter and whipped butter is ideal for this treatment. These will provide extra nourishment for the skin. You can customize this treatment with other essential oils if preferred.

Supplies needed:

- 1 plush or fleece blanket
- 1 mylar blanket (optional) for extra heat
- 1-2 large bath towels
- 2 Twin flat sheets
- Pillowcase for breast draping
- Dry brush or exfoliating gloves
- Your oil or butter blend

Precautions:

- This treatment is ideal for clients who want to enhance massage results, relax deep tension, improve skin appearance, and those who feel cold.
- Do not perform on claustrophobic or easily overheated clients, children, or those with skin disorders without doctor clearance.
- This treatment is not for weight loss.

Cocoon Layers (in order):

- Client lays between 2 flat sheets
- Table warmer
- Fitted sheet
- Flat sheet
- (Optional) Mylar blanket
- Flat sheet
- Plush blanket

Application (beginning prone):

- Dry brush each limb toward the heart.
- Dry brush entire back.
- Apply product over entire body while prone.
- Have client turn supine.
- Dry brush limbs toward heart.
- Drape breasts with pillowcase for female clients.
- Dry brush abdomen clockwise.
- Dry brush pecs gently toward armpits.
- Apply product over entire body while supine.

Cocooning:

- Have the client place hands in a position where they will be comfortable for at least 20 minutes.
- Fold blanket over starting at shoulders.
- Crisscross corners of sheet over chest, then slip each blanket layer over right side and then left to form a "burrito".
- Add the last layer of a thick blanket on top for warmth.

Relaxation:

- Provide eye pillow or mask and let client relax with warmth for 20-30 minutes, periodically checking comfort.

Enhancements:

- While the client is wrapped, add facial and scalp massage.
- Note: You may also place a warm rice pack over the abdomen or incorporate a castor oil pack.

Scalp Treatments

Nourishing scalp treatments feel luxurious and can be an add on to any treatment. They are therapeutic and help relieve tension. As you massage the oils into the scalp, the client receives the deeply relaxing benefits from inhaling the essential oils. Gua Sha combs are available to facilitate the distribution of the scalp oil in combination with massage.

The client can leave it on for an hour and then wash off or leave it on until the next day.

Carrier Oils beneficial for scalp treatments: argan oil, jojoba oil, almond oil, coconut oil, pumpkin seed oil, and castor oil.

Essential Oils that are beneficial for scalp treatments:

- Rosemary Essential Oil: Stimulates blood circulation to the scalp, promotes hair thickness, and is anti-fungal.
- Lavender Essential Oil: Promotes hair growth, soothes the scalp, and has antimicrobial properties that can help with dandruff.
- Peppermint Essential Oil: Refreshes the scalp, increases circulation, and may help with hair growth and thickness.
- Tea Tree Essential Oil: Antimicrobial and anti-inflammatory. Can help with dandruff, scalp acne, and other scalp conditions.
- Cedarwood Essential Oil: Balances oil production, stimulates hair follicles, and can help with hair loss and thinning.
- Ylang Ylang Essential Oil: Promotes hair growth, balances sebum production, possesses antimicrobial properties, and offers a soothing and calming effect.

- Bergamot Essential Oil: contains compounds that may stimulate/invigorate the hair follicles and promote hair growth, regulates sebum production and has antibacterial and antifungal properties.

Scalp Oil Recipes

Combine the carrier oils and essential oils in a clean, dark-colored glass bottle. Apply a small amount of the scalp oil blend to the scalp and gently massage it in using circular motions. Leave it on for at least 30 minutes, or overnight if preferred, before shampooing as usual. Use regularly for best results.

Balancing Scalp Oil Blend:

- 2 tablespoons Argan Oil
- 1 tablespoon Almond Oil
- 5 drops Bergamot Essential Oil
- 5 drops Ylang Ylang Essential Oil
- 3 drops Cedarwood Essential Oil

Hair Growth Stimulating Scalp Oil:

- 2 tablespoons Coconut Oil
- 1 tablespoon Jojoba Oil
- 5 drops Rosemary Essential Oil
- 5 drops Lavender Essential Oil
- 3 drops Cedarwood Essential Oil

Soothing Scalp Relief Blend:

- 2 tablespoons Almond Oil
- 1 tablespoon Jojoba Oil
- 5 drops Lavender Essential Oil
- 5 drops Bergamot Essential Oil
- 3 drops Ylang Ylang Essential Oil

Nourishing and Strengthening Scalp Oil:

- 2 tablespoons Argan Oil
- 1 tablespoon Coconut Oil
- 5 drops Cedarwood Essential Oil
- 5 drops Rosemary Essential Oil
- 3 drops Ylang Ylang Essential Oil

Scalp Rejuvenating Oil Blend:

- 2 tablespoons Jojoba Oil
- 1 tablespoon Almond Oil
- 5 drops Bergamot Essential Oil
- 5 drops Lavender Essential Oil
- 3 drops Rosemary Essential Oil

'What comes from the heart, touches the heart" **-Don Sibet**

Your Aromatherapy Practice

Your Scope

As bodyworkers, we do not diagnose conditions or prescribe treatments; that falls within a physician's scope of practice. However, we can offer information and resources to support individuals in conducting their own research, enabling them to make informed decisions regarding their medical and wellness care.

This includes education on contraindications and the safe and proper way to use essential oils.

If you don't know the answer, it's ok to say "I'm not sure, but I will find out."

Create a list of educational resources that you can have in your pocket to reference and share with clients.

Do you need a separate intake form?

Ultimately, the decision is yours. It's customary for massage therapists and bodyworkers to employ a health history form prior to administering treatments to clients. Similarly, these intake forms are applicable for aromatherapy-based bodywork sessions.

Consider adding a few questions to your existing intake form that will help you when creating a custom treatment:

Do you have any favorite essential oils?

- o   Are there any aromas that you dislike?
- o   Do you have any allergies to nuts, seeds, or other vegetable oils?
- o   Do you have any known allergies to different aromas?

Bodywork Applications

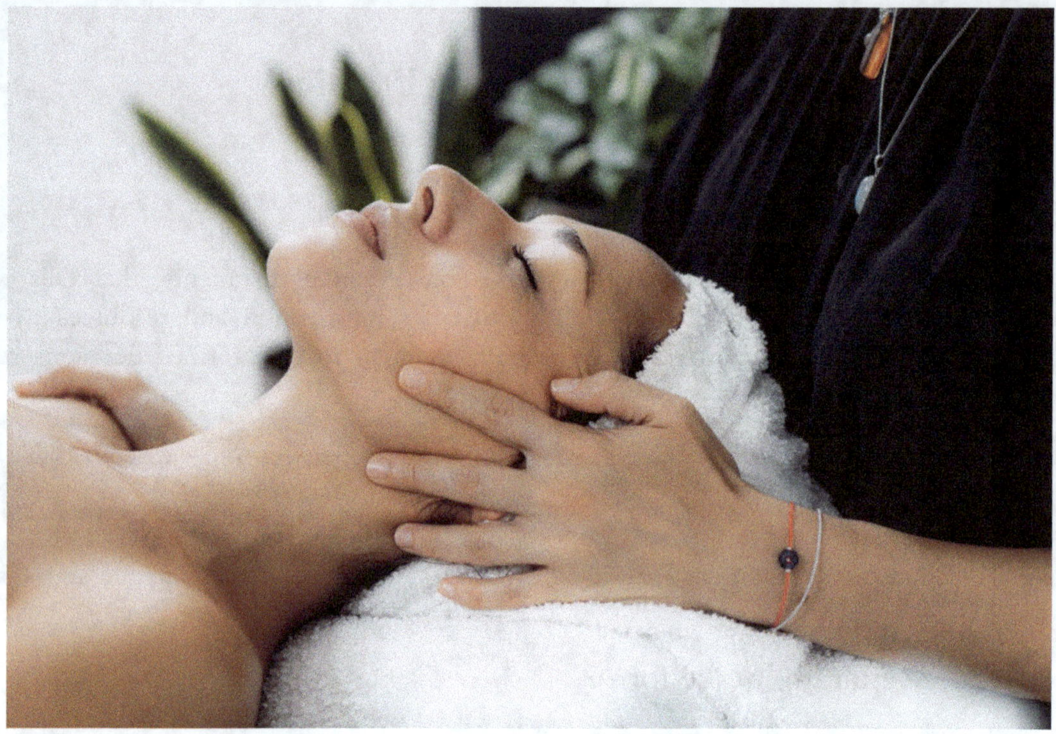

Aromatherapy complements various modalities and styles of bodywork, potentially enhancing the results of any session.

Whether you're doing pure relaxation or more of a focused "treatment" such as in Neuromuscular Therapy or Sports Massage—weaving in botanical formulas and aromatherapy tools will enhance the overall goals for the session.

Reflexology

Reflexology and aromatherapy complement each other so well because they use an alternative lens through which to view healing. Reflexologists focus on affecting both the energetic and physical body of the person through nerve endings on different points of the feet.

You can choose an oil or a blend based custom for your client and give them a more holistic and profound healing experience with you.

> Pro tip: Have a warm castor oil pack on hand for your reflexology clients to lie on their abdomen, since they are supine during the session.

Treatment Focused - Clinical Massage, NMT, Sports, MFR, etc.

These sessions are usually focused on treating chronic or acute complaints like back or neck pain, pulled muscles, spasms, inflammation, and other muscular injuries.

Utilizing muscle balms, gels, salves, or blends with higher dilutions (e.g., 5-10%) can significantly enhance the effectiveness of these treatments. Higher concentrations are indicated for smaller areas or "spot treatments" to assist with the above. You can also have a lower dilution blend (e.g., 2-3%) to work on larger areas.

My favorite oils for treatment focused bodywork include: Rosemary, Juniper, Peppermint, Ginger, Black Pepper, Clary Sage, Copaiba, Turmeric and Basil.

Relaxation Focused

When your client simply wants to decompress, rest, and relax. Relaxation massage is also indicated for people who have overtaxed nervous systems or grappling with conditions such as anxiety, depression, or PTSD.

Which oils come to mind when you think of soothing and comforting? I think of Lavender, Chamomile, Orange, Geranium, Mandarin, Clary Sage, Vetiver, Bergamot, Frankincense, Yarrow, and Ylang Ylang.

Perhaps a mist of hydrosol can make for a lovely opening or closing to a session.

Manual Lymphatic Drainage

If you are certified in MLD, consider using essential oils with an affinity for the lymphatic system in your treatment.

A lower dilution is appropriate as you are covering larger areas of the body. 1-3%

Castor oil packs are ideal for use during these types of treatments.

Oils with an affinity for the lymphatic system:

- Lime
- Orange
- Grapefruit
- Juniper
- Cypress
- Rosemary
- Scotch Pine
- Calendula Infused herb oil

Facial Massage

Aromatics can significantly enhance facial massage by offering a multi-dimensional approach to relaxation and rejuvenation. Firstly, as we apply the oils to the facial region, the recipient will benefit from the direct impact the essential oils have on the mind, promoting a sense of calm and reducing stress and anxiety during the massage session. This mental relaxation can contribute to a more enjoyable and effective massage experience.

Certain essential oils possess potent anti-inflammatory properties, which can help reduce redness, swelling, and irritated skin. When incorporated into facial massage, these oils can ease tension and puffiness, resulting in a smoother and more radiant complexion.

Many vegetable carrier oils are renowned for their beneficial effects on skin health. They can hydrate, nourish, and protect the skin, promoting elasticity and suppleness while combating signs of aging. By infusing the massage experience with these skin-loving oils, facial massage becomes not only a luxurious treat but also a treatment for maintaining healthy and vibrant skin.

- Use a .5-1% dilution when formulating blends for the facial region.
- Avoid dermal irritants. Use only gentle essential oils on the face.
- Carrier Oils that are beneficial for the facial region include: Argan oil, Apricot oil, Camellia oil and Jojoba wax.
- Gentle essential oils include: Chamomile, Lavender, Geranium, Clary Sage, Ylang Ylang, Palmarosa, Copaiba, Frankincense, and Vetiver.

Cupping and Gua Sha

Applying oils can be comforting and also reinforce the benefits of the treatments. In my practice, I have successfully incorporated the use of topical botanicals, including herbal-infused oils, essential oil blends, and herbal balms, following cupping or Gua Sha treatments. I feel it may contribute to the fact that the pores are more open and ready to receive this therapeutic application. It also feels soothing and comforting after these "intense" treatments.

Barefoot Massage (Ashiatsu)

When performing barefoot modalities, grip is important. You can enhance the session with the benefits of aromatics by using a massage butter (e.g. the whipped butter or the subtle shea soft butter) and adding the appropriate amount of essential oils for the goals and intentions of the treatment.

Body Brushing (Dry Skin Brushing)

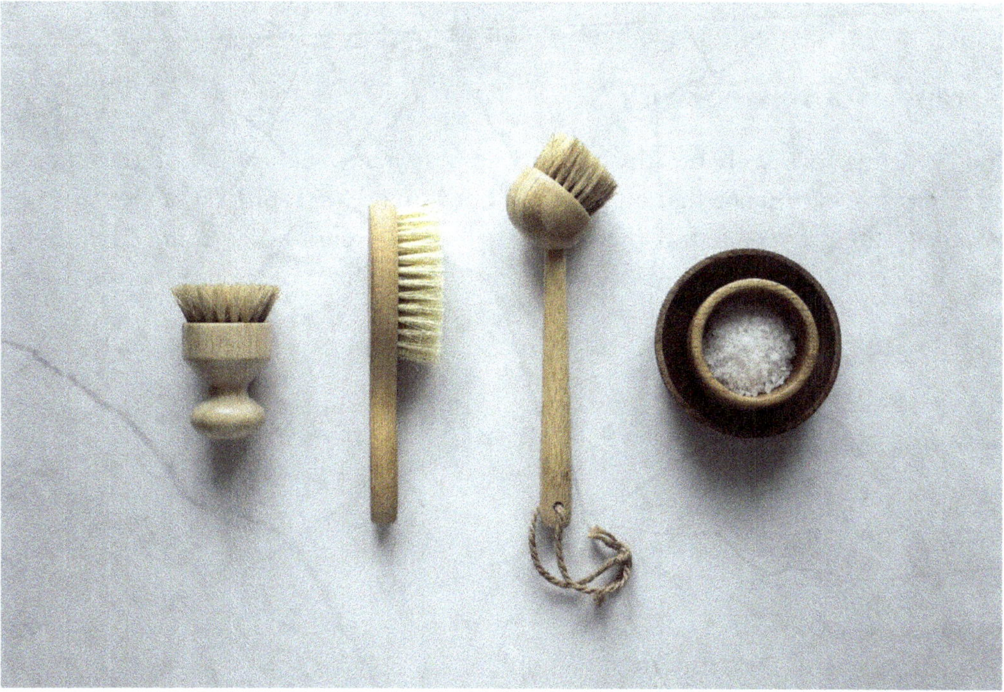

Dry skin brushing is very popular in the east and has become popular all over the world in spas and as a home self-care beauty ritual. Not only does it sloth off dead skin cells, it also stimulates circulation and lymphatic drainage.

All you need is a natural wooden bristle brush. Strokes should be light, and when working on the extremities, in the direction toward the heart. Be sure to not brush too hard and check on the comfort level of the client. Dry brushing should be performed while the skin is dry. Once you have finished the body brushing while the client is prone and supine, you may now proceed with your massage using oils and/or body wraps.

Always prioritize the client's well-being, adapting the brushing technique based on individual preferences and sensitivities.

To body brush a client:

Instruct the client to disrobe and lie face down on the massage table, covering themselves with a towel or sheet for modesty.

1. Begin dry brushing by gently brushing the client's back and shoulders using long, sweeping strokes. Working from the spin outward, down and up the back, ect.
2. Move to the arms, legs, feet, and hands, continuing with the same technique, paying attention to brush towards the heart.

3. Be mindful of sensitive areas and adjust pressure accordingly. Communicate with the client to ensure they are comfortable throughout the process.
4. You may now start your treatment, whether it's a massage with oil or body wrap.

Aromatherapy and Breathe work

Incorporating essential oils with breathwork can amplify the benefits of both practices, offering a holistic and immersive experience that nurtures the body, mind, and spirit. Whether seeking relaxation, focus, emotional support, respiratory health, or enhanced mind-body connection, the synergistic combination of essential oils and breathwork provides a powerful tool for holistic wellness.

Benefits Include:

- Enhanced Relaxation
- Heightened Focus and Clarity
- Emotional Support
- Respiratory Support
- Mind-Body Connection

Square Breathing and Aromatherapy

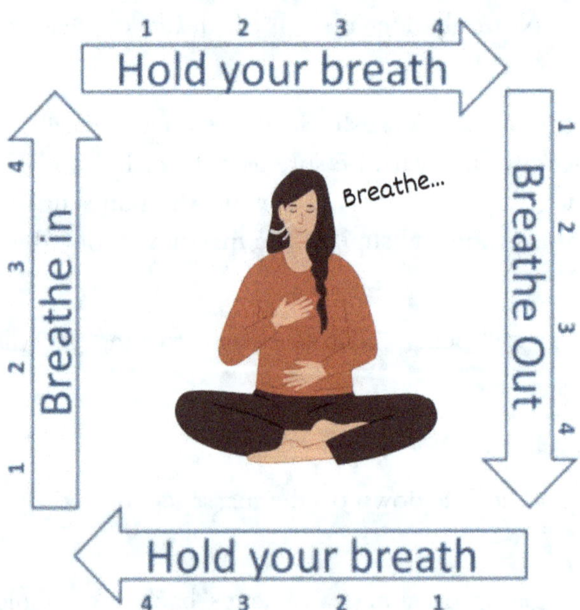

Square breathing, also known as box breathing, is a simple and effective technique for managing anxiety and promoting relaxation. It involves four equal steps, each corresponding to a specific count of inhalation, hold, exhalation, and hold. The exercise below can help you recenter, no matter if you are at work, home, or on the go. Do it with your aromatherapy inhaler. Square breathing can help calm the nervous system, reduce feelings of anxiety, and promote a sense of relaxation and centeredness, while improving focus and concentration: This technique involves mind + body at the same time. It is a great stress buster! You can feel the calmness just after doing this exercise.

Repeat these four steps in a continuous cycle, maintaining a steady rhythm and focusing your attention on the sensations of your breath:

1. Inhale (Count to 4): Begin by taking a slow, deep breath through your nose, counting to four as you fill your lungs with air. Focus on breathing deeply into your diaphragm, allowing your abdomen to expand.
2. Hold (Count to 4): Once you have completed the inhalation, hold your breath for a count of four. Maintain a comfortable and relaxed state during this brief pause, keeping your focus on your breath.
3. Exhale (Count to 4): Slowly release the breath through your mouth, counting to four as you exhale. Empty your lungs completely, allowing any tension or stress to leave your body with each breath out.
4. Hold (Count to 4): After exhaling, pause for another count of four before beginning the next inhalation. Use this moment to relax and prepare for the next cycle of breathing.

Seasonal Blends

These are a great way to keep things fresh in your practice. They can be tailored to align with the current season's events. For example, in spring when people are out gardening and straining their backs, how about choosing blends that help alleviate pain? Other examples include cooling blends for summer and warming blends for winter. Be creative!

Eye Pillows

While the client is supine, the therapist can use a folded washcloth or eye pillow with a drop of oil such as Lavender or Eucalyptus to promote relaxation and open the breath. The light pressure, combined with blocking out light and the inhalation of aromatic essences, helps lower stress levels and supports deep relaxation.

How do you plan to integrate Aromatherapy into your practice?

Essential Oil Quick Guide

This is your cheat sheet that you can use for quick reference anytime.

Analgesic: Alleviates or diminishes pain: pain-relieving, for mild and severe pain, chronic or acute, for shoulder pain, muscle or joint pain, etc.: Rosemary, Basil, Bay Laurel, Bergamot, Black Pepper, Clary sage, clove, German Chamomile, Eucalyptus radiata, Fir, Geranium, Ginger, Juniper Berry, Lavender, Lemongrass, Marjoram, Niaouli, Peppermint, Tea Tree.

Antidepressant: Uplifting to the mood, helpful for depressive states: An agent that is uplifting and counteracts melancholy: Bergamot, Basil, Clary Sage, Geranium, Ginger, Grapefruit, Jasmine, Lavender, Lime, Lemongrass, Litsea Cubeba, Mandarin, Orange, Patchouli, Rose, Rosemary, Ylang Ylang

Anti-fungal or fungicidal: inhibits and destroys fungi and mold growth: Basil, German Chamomile, Clary Sage, Helichrysum, Geranium, Lemongrass, Marjoram, Patchouli, Peppermint, Ravensara, Rosemary, Spearmint, Spruce, Tea Tree

Anti-infectious: An agent that is capable of acting against infection: Basil, Bay Laurel, Bergamot, Eucalyptus radiata, Helichrysum, Fennel, Geranium, Lavender, Lemon, Lemongrass, Litsea Cubeba, Marjoram, Niaouli, Patchouli, Pine, Ravensara, Rosemary, Rose, Spruce, Tea Tree, Thyme

Anti-inflammatory: helps to reduce and prevent inflammation: Basil, German Chamomile, Helichrysum, Fennel, Geranium, Lavender, Litsea Cubeba, Niaouli, Patchouli, Peppermint, Ravensara, Rosemary, Rose, Spearmint, Spruce, Tea Tree

Antispasmodic: An agent that prevents and eases spasms and relieves cramps: Basil, Black Pepper, German Chamomile, Cinnamon, Clary Sage, Cypress, Eucalyptus radiata, Helichrysum, Fennel, Geranium, Jasmine, Juniper Berry, Lavender, Lemon, Mandarin, Marjoram,Orange, Peppermint, Rose, Spearmint, Spruce, Thyme

Antiseptic: Cleansing oils that prevent the development of microbes: Basil, Bay Laurel, Bergamot, Black Pepper, Cardamom, Cedarwood, Cinnamon, Cypress, Helichrysum, Fir, Frankincense, Geranium, Ginger, Jasmine, Juniper Berry, Lavender, Lemongrass, Litsea Cubeba, Marjoram, Niaouli, Patchouli, Peppermint, Pine, Ravensara, Rose, Spearmint, Tea Tree, Thyme, Vetiver, Ylang Ylang

Aphrodisiac: this increases sexual desire or excitement. An agent that provokes sexual interest and excitement: Ylang Ylang, Amyris, Ginger, Cinnamon, Jasmine, Rose, Patchouli.

Astringent: These contract, tighten and tone blood vessels and body tissue: Cedarwood, Cypress, Eucalyptus radiata, Frankincense, Geranium, Juniper Berry, Lavender, Lemon, Lemongrass, Litsea Cubeba, Patchouli, Peppermint, Rosemary,

Calming: These oils calm the mind and promote a tranquilizing/pacifying effect, reduces anxiety, nervousness, distress, or agitation: Cedarwood, Chamomile (Roman & German), Clary Sage, Geranium, Jasmine, Jatamansi Lavender, Mandarin, Marjoram, Myrrh, Orange, Vetiver, Ylang Ylang,

Carminative: this reduces intestinal spasm, settles the digestive system. An agent that settles the digestive system and the expulsion of gas from the intestines: Basil, Bay Laurel, Bergamot, Black Pepper, Cardamom, German Chamomile, Cinnamon, Fennel, Frankincense, Geranium, Ginger, Juniper Berry, Lavender, Lemon, Lemongrass, Litsea Cubeba, Marjoram, Orange, Peppermint, Rosemary, Thyme

Cicatrizant: promotes healing of scar tissue: Helichrysum, Frankincense, Bergamot, German Chamomile, Eucalyptus radiata, Lemon, Niaouli, Patchouli, Rosemary, Rose, Spearmint, Tea Tree, Thyme

Cephalic: this is stimulating and clears the mind: Rosemary, Basil, Cardamom, Peppermint, Spearmint, Lime, Bergamot, Eucalyptus globulus

Decongestant: this reduces or relieves congestion: German Chamomile, Clary Sage, Eucalyptus radiata, Fennel, Geranium, Grapefruit, Juniper Berry, Lavender, Lemon, Mandarin, Marjoram, Niaouli, Orange, Patchouli, Peppermint, Ravensara, Rosemary, Rose

Deodorant: this destroys or inhibits odors: Bergamot, Clary Sage, Cypress, Eucalyptus radiata, Fir, Geranium, Lavender, Lemongrass, Patchouli, Pine

Detoxifying: these oils help to stimulate lymph and fluid movement in the body, supporting movement of impurities and liver and kidney energy: Juniper, Rosemary, Cypress, Grapefruit, Mandarin, Lemon, Lime, Bergamot, Orange, Laurel.

Digestive: this aids the digestion of food: Basil, Bay Laurel, Cardamom, German Chamomile, Helichrysum, Fennel, Lavender, Mandarin, Marjoram, Niaouli, Orange, Peppermint, Rosemary, Rose

Diuretic: this aids urine production: Cardamom, Cedarwood, Cypress, Eucalyptus radiata, Helichrysum, Fennel, Frankincense, Geranium, Grapefruit, Mandarin, Patchouli, Pine, Rosemary, Thyme

Expectorant: this expels mucus in the respiratory system: Basil, Bay Laurel, Cardamom, Cedarwood, Eucalyptus radiata, Helichrysum, Fir, Frankincense, Ginger, Marjoram, Niaouli, Peppermint, Pine, Ravensara, Tea Tree, Thyme

Euphoric: Elation or intense state of happiness and feelings of wellbeing: Bergamot, Clary Sage, Copaiba, Myrrh, Nutmeg, Ylang Ylang, Grapefruit, Jasmine, Frankincense, Rose Otto, neroli.

Febrifuge: helps reduce fever with cooling properties that reduce high body temperature: Basil, Bay Laurel, Bergamot, Black Pepper, Eucalyptus radiata, Ginger, Lemon, Lemongrass, Niaouli, Patchouli, Peppermint, Spruce

Immune stimulant: supports a healthy function of the immune system: Cypress, Frankincense, Niaouli, Patchouli, Tea Tree

Hormone influencer: A tonic for the endocrine system: Basil, German Chamomile, Clary Sage, Helichrysum, Fennel, Geranium, Juniper Berry, Marjoram, Niaouli, Peppermint, Rosemary, Spruce, Ylang Ylang

Rubefacient: this is warming and increases blood flow: Black Pepper, Clove, Eucalyptus radiata, Fir, Ginger, Orange, Niaouli, Pine, Rosemary, Turmeric, Vetiver

Sedative: Promotes restful sleep, calms the mind, lessens excitement: Cedarwood, German & Roman Chamomile, Clary Sage, Frankincense, Jasmine, Jatamansi, Lavender, Mandarin, Marjoram, Myrrh, Orange, Patchouli, Rose, Valerian, Vetiver, Ylang Ylang

Stimulant: These have an energizing and uplifting effect on the body and mind by stimulating the physiological functions of the body: Rosemary, Basil, Cardamom, Cinnamon, Fir, Ginger, Grapefruit, Juniper Berry, Litsea Cubeba, Niaouli, Peppermint, , Spearmint, Tea Tree, Thyme

Tonic: strengthens and enlivens the body or parts of the body: Basil, Bay Laurel, Bergamot, Cardamom, Clary Sage, Cypress, Helichrysum, Fennel, Ginger, Juniper Berry, Lemon, Litsea Cubeba, Marjoram, Niaouli, Pine, Ravensara, Rosemary, Rose, Spearmint, Spruce, Thyme, Vetiver

Vulnerary: promotes healing of wounds: Bergamot, German Chamomile, Eucalyptus radiata, Frankincense, Geranium, Juniper Berry, Lavender, Marjoram, Niaouli

Measurements and Dilutions

Dilution Chart

Carrier Oil in ounces	0.5% Dilution	1%	2.5%	3%	5%	10%
10 ml (Roll-on)	1 drop	2 drops	3 drops	6 drops	10 drops	20 drops
½ ounce (15ml)	1-2 drops	3 drops	7-8 drops	9 drops	15 drops	30 drops
1 ounce (30ml)	3 drops	6 drops	15 drops	18 drops	30 drops	60 drops
2 ounces (60 ml)	6 drops	12 drops	30 drops	36 drops	60 drops	120 drops
4 ounces (120ml)	12 drops	24 drops	60 drops	72 drops	120 drops	240 drops

- **1% Dilution** — Use for children (under 12) pregnant women and people with long-term illnesses or immune system disorders. A 1% dilution is also a good place to start with individuals who are generally sensitive to chemicals, fragrances, or other environmental pollutants.
- **2% Dilution** — Use for general wellness supporting products such as bath oils, skin care, natural perfumes, or for blends you like to use on a daily basis.
- **3% Dilution** — Use this dilution when creating a blend to address a specific, acute health concern, such as pain relief or getting through a cold or flu.
- **5% Dilution-** Used for addressing acute conditions and for localized treatments.
- **10% Dilution-** Indicated when stronger effect is needed for acute muscular aches and pains, Trauma injury, treatment massage, and localized treatment work, muscle balms and salves.

Measurement Cart

How many drops in an ounce or ml? This chart can help you when formulating your blends on the go or when making larger batches.

1ml	20 drops			
5mls	100 drops	1 teaspoon		
10mls	200 drops	2 teaspoons	1/3 ounce	
15mls	300 drops	1 tablespoon	½ ounce	
30mls	600 drops	2 tablespoons	1 ounce	
60mls	1200 drops	4 tablespoons	2 ounces	
120mls	2400 drops	8 tablespoons	4 ounces	½ cup
240mls	3600 drops	16 tablespoons	8 ounces	1 cup

Glossary - The Language // Botanical Talk

Analgesic: oils used to reduce pain.

Antiseptics/Anti-microbial: prevent the growth of bacteria and resist pathogenic microorganisms.

Anti-spasmodic: prevent or ease cramps in the body and muscle spasms.

Astringents: shrink or constrict body tissues.

Carminative: stimulate the peristalsis of the digestive system and help ease digestion by relieving gas, spasms and cramps.

Cephalic: of or relating to the head.

Dermal sensitization: is a type of allergic reaction. Occurs with subsequent exposure to the same material over a long period of time.

Dermal irritants: will cause an immediate inflammatory reaction when applied to the skin.

Diaphoretics: induces sweating.

Emmenagogue: Herbs that help promote menstruation flow and bring on the cycle.

Emollient: softens and soothes the skin and mucous membranes.

Exfoliant: a mechanical or chemical agent (such as an abrasive skin wash or salicylic acid) that is applied to the skin to remove dead cells from the surface.

Expectorant: Promotes the discharge or expulsion of mucus from the respiratory tract.

Humectant: a substance that promotes retention of moisture.

Neat: Used undiluted.

Hydrophobic: Water repelling, not soluble in water.

Nervines: calm, strengthen and tone the nervous system.

Lipophilic: Oil soluble, attracted to fat, water insoluble.

Rubefacient: a substance that increases cutaneous blood flow to a local area; causes reddening and warming of the skin.

Sedative: Reduce stress and nervous disorders throughout the body. They serve as aids for sleep and to promote calmness.

Solvent: the substance used to dissolve the chemical constituents of another substance.

Stimulants: Increase the energy of the body by quickening and enlivening the physiological function of the body.

Volatile: Substance volatility refers to the ability of an essential oil to turn from liquid to vapor.

Vulnerary: help heal the body by promoting cell growth and repair; Used in the healing of wounds.

About the Author

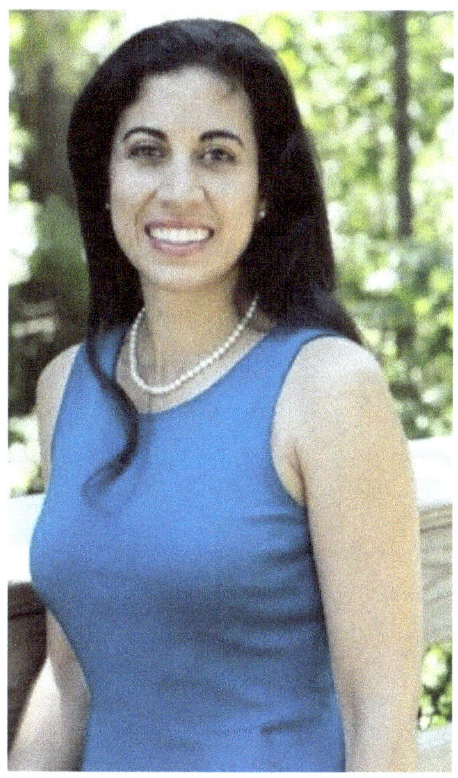

Fernanda Santiago, born in the vibrant Island of Puerto Rico, embodies a lineage steeped in the art of natural healing. Descended from a lineage of midwives and herbalists, Fernanda's roots run deep in the traditions of holistic wellness. Her great grandmother, revered for her expertise in natural healing compounds, passed down a legacy of herbal medicine and holistic practices through generations.

With an innate passion for wellness and a desire to aid others on their journey to health, Fernanda embarked on a path dedicated to Aromatic Botanical Medicine over two decades ago. Her journey led her to Chiang Mai, Thailand, where she delved into the intricate world of natural healing under the guidance of Acupuncture Physicians and Botanists, gaining invaluable hands-on experience along the way.

Formally trained by esteemed Aromatherapy schools, Fernanda's expertise in Aromatherapy is matched only by her commitment to holistic wellness. She has cultivated her skills and knowledge through her private practice, Healing Feels Good®, nestled in the serene town of Apex, NC. Here, she provides personalized consultations, Aromatherapy treatments, and bespoke formulations, complemented by rejuvenating bodywork sessions including Reflexology, Thai Massage, and Thai Herbal Poultice treatments.

As a co-founder of Apex Retreat Seminars, Fernanda extends her passion for education, establishing a nationally approved continuing education school tailored for massage therapists. Recognized as a Certified Professional Aromatherapist, Fernanda's dedication to her craft is evident in her unwavering commitment to sharing her wisdom and traditional healing methods with others.

Driven by a love for gardening, a connection to the outdoors, and a fervent desire to empower others on their wellness journey, Fernanda Santiago stands as a beacon of holistic healing, bridging the gap between tradition and modernity with every formulation, treatment, and consultation she offers.

www.ingramcontent.com/pod-product-compliance
Lightning Source LLC
Chambersburg PA
CBHW060510120726
48002CB00011B/3104